The Veterinarian's Companion
for
Common Dental
PROCEDURES

The Veterinarian's Companion
for
Common Dental
PROCEDURES

Heidi B. Lobprise, DVM
Diplomate, American Veterinary Dental College
Associate, Dallas Dental Service Animal Clinic

Robert B. Wiggs, DVM
Diplomate, American Veterinary Dental College
Director, Dallas Dental Service Animal Clinic
Associate Adjunct Professor, Baylor College of Dentistry, Texas A & M
University System

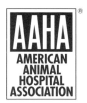

AAHA®
AMERICAN
ANIMAL
HOSPITAL
ASSOCIATION

Many thanks to the AAHA Press Editorial Advisory Board:
Dr. Laurel Collins, ABVP
Dr. Richard Goebel
Dr. Charles Hickey
Dr. Clayton McKinnon
Dr. Richard Nelson, ABVP
Dr. Hal Taylor

The authors would also like to acknowledge and thank Dr. Michael Peak for his assistance in the review and preparation of this book.

Unless otherwise noted, all illustrations in this volume are provided by R. B. Wiggs.

AAHA Press
12575 W. Bayaud Avenue
Lakewood, Colorado 80228

ISBN 1-58326-006-4

Contents

Chapter 1 — Oral Anatomy and Physiology   1

Chapter 2 — Oral Examination and Recognition of Pathology   11

Chapter 4 — Oral Surgery   71

Illustrations

PLATES

FIGURES

TABLES

Introduction

A lecturer once told a story about a client who asked if he really had to brush his pet's teeth, to which the veterinarian replied, "Only those teeth you want to save." That correlation can also be made on a practice level. If you ask yourself which clients you should approach with recommendations for a strong oral hygiene program and dental education, the response would be, "Only those who care for their pets." There are certainly individual clients who will never be receptive to veterinary care that extends beyond the bare necessities, but by offering proper education about the oral and systemic benefits of dental care, you can provide the best care possible for those who wish to give their pets all they can.

And let's face it, dentistry is here to stay! Although you might not get to use that new endoscope or ultrasound unit on every patient, each animal who comes through your door has a mouth, and the great majority of your patients already have some degree of periodontal disease, not to mention broken teeth, malocclusions, and on and on.

This text is designed to serve the general population of pets that enter veterinarians' offices each day. We organized the information by sticking to the "meat and potatoes" of veterinary dentistry, emphasizing areas we regularly encounter with our own patients and those we discuss with other veterinarians who call or come by with questions.

A large percentage of veterinarians practicing today were given no formal training in the field of dentistry. Fortunately, many avenues are open today for those who wish to continue their education in this area, and several good books are available. In this volume, we provide a readily available, "user-friendly" handbook that can be consulted on a daily basis. We have compiled a basic background of anatomy and pathology primarily related to clinical situations and then covered most of the oral and dental problems you might encounter, together with treatment options. Situations that call for more advanced treatment modalities, such as endodontics and orthodontics, are addressed as well to help you recognize situations in which such modalities are indicated as well as patients who need to be referred or treated with other options. However, the main focus of this book is on common dental procedures.

Our goal was to offer you the basic information of our field and encourage the development of fundamental skills that will result in better oral, dental, and even systemic health for your patients. Most of the general information, from anatomical considerations to disease processes and treatment, apply to dogs and cats, with specific differences noted. There is also a chapter devoted specifically to pocket pets. It is our hope that, through your use of this book, your patients will benefit, your clients will appreciate your services, and your practice will grow as well.

If you are interested in furthering your veterinary dental education, we urge you to join the American Veterinary Dental Society (AVDS), which publishes the *Journal of Veterinary Dentistry* on a quarterly basis (call 1-800-332-AVDS). Informative articles, details on upcoming meetings (including the Annual Veterinary Dental Forum), and other valuable resources can be found in the journal, and the AVDS promotes participation in activities that enhance veterinary dentistry on all levels, among them National Pet Dental Health Month.

We have also provided additional reference materials and a recommended reading list for those of you who would like more information about veterinary dentistry.

CHAPTER 1

Oral Anatomy and Physiology

It is important to be able to recognize the normal anatomical features of the oral cavity and understand the typical physiological processes that occur there. This chapter will highlight clinically significant areas of oral anatomy and physiology and point out the ways in which they are relevant to clinical practice.

OSSEOUS ANATOMY

Teeth are, of course, the most visually prominent features of the mouth, and typically, they are the first to be examined. However, the osseous structures, which play an essential role in supporting the teeth, warrant careful examination as well. The formation, structure, and preservation of the bones of the head and face can greatly influence dental integrity and *occlusion* (Figure 1.1).

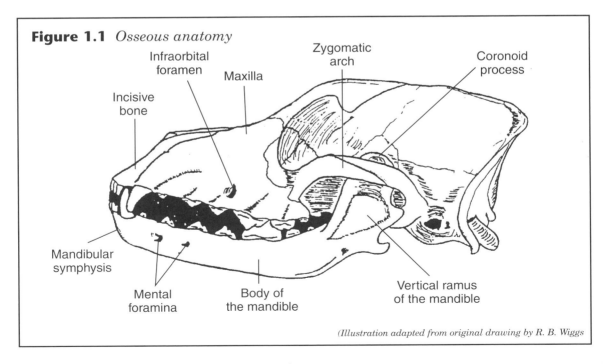

Figure 1.1 *Osseous anatomy*

Infraorbital foramen

Zygomatic arch

Coronoid process

Maxilla

Incisive bone

Mandibular symphysis

Mental foramina

Body of the mandible

Vertical ramus of the mandible

(Illustration adapted from original drawing by R. B. Wiggs

Maxillae

Teeth are housed in the *alveolar sockets* found in the jaws. The hard tissue of the upper jaw and palate is formed by three bones: the single, u-shaped *incisive bone* located rostrally and the paired *maxillae* (right and left). The two sides of the maxilla are joined at the midline and are rostrally attached to the incisive bone, making a y-shaped suture line. Defects in the fusing of these bones and associated soft tissue result in clefts. A midline defect behind the incisive bone is called a *secondary palatal cleft,* and one between the incisive bone and maxillae is called a *primary palatal cleft* or *cleft lip* if the lip is involved. The incisors are located in the incisive bone, and the remaining teeth are in the maxillae.

The buccal cortical bone of the maxillae is fairly thin, allowing adequate palpation of the *alveolar juga,* or protrusions where maxillae tooth roots are located. The rostral opening of the infraorbital canal can be palpated dorsal to the upper fourth premolars, at the point where the vessels and nerves exit. The canal is situated very close to the two *mesial* (rostral) roots of the tooth, so in doing any surgical work in the region, you should avoid those structures. Likewise, whenever possible, the large palatine arteries, located on either side of the palate and running in the palatine grooves, should be avoided.

Mandibles

The paired mandibles have three regions: the symphysis, the body, and the vertical ramus. The pair are joined at the symphysis rostrally; the joint they form is sometimes fibrous and has some degree of movement. Other than the *incisors* in the symphyseal region, all other teeth (*canines, premolars,* and *molars*) are housed in the body of the mandible. The mandibular canal runs the length of the body of the mandible, just ventral to the tooth roots, and *mental foramina* allow the exit of vessels from the canal to supply rostral structures. Both the canal and the foramina will appear as lucencies on radiographs.

The *condyloid process* at the distal aspect of the mandibular vertical ramus articulates with the mandibular fossa of the temporal bone as the *temporomandibular joint* (TMJ). The flat *coronoid process* lies medial to the *zygomatic arch.*

Alveoli

The *alveoli,* or bony sockets, are the structures that specifically house the *roots* of the teeth. The jaws have a dense cortical bone covering the trabecular bone, and the *alveolar bone* is also a dense cortical bone, often seen as the *lamina dura* on radiographs. The interdental cortical bone, or the *alveolar crest,* is often the first area affected with bone loss during periodontal disease.

ORAL SOFT TISSUE

The soft tissue of the oral cavity provides cover and protection for the osseous tissue and aids in the support of the teeth and the function of the oral cavity. The earliest changes in the oral cavity often affect the soft tissue, as seen, for example, in gingival inflammation. This tissue can also reflect systemic diseases, such as anemia, cyanosis, and even uremia (with systemic uremia, the soft tissues of the mouth may be ulcerated).

Tongue

The tongue is formed mainly of skeletal muscle, with intrinsic and extrinsic muscles that work together to provide the complicated movements necessary for prehension, swallowing, and grooming. The tongue is divided into the tip, the margins, the body (where most taste buds are located), and the root. The tongue is connected to the floor of the mouth at the rostral extent by the lingual *frenulum,* near which salivary ducts (mandibular, sublingual) open at the sublingual caruncles.

Palate

The *palate,* or roof of the mouth, is covered by keratinized epithelium and typically is characterized by *rugae,* or rugal folds. The *incisive papilla* is a mound of tissue found behind the upper incisors and is the exit site for the vomeronasal ducts, which are part of the vomeronasal organ.

Lips

Lips form at the junction of the buccal mucosa and adjacent skin on the outside. They close to help protect the oral cavity and are often used in food prehension. Further attachment of the lips is enhanced by frenula (paired near the mandibular canines and single midline at the rostral maxillae). Excessive tension exerted by the lips at the site of frenulum attachment can exacerbate periodontal inflammation.

Muscles of Mastication

Most of the muscles of mastication, including the largest temporalis muscle (which arises from temporal fossa) and the masseter muscle (arising from the zygomatic arch), insert on the mandibles and act to close the jaws. The digastric muscle, arising from the jugular process of the occipital bone and inserting on the ventral border of the mandible, helps to open the mouth. These strong muscles give a powerful biting force, although atrophy or myositis in the muscles can greatly inhibit normal chewing behavior.

Salivary Glands

Salivary glands produce saliva to play a role in oral lubrication and food digestion. In the dog, the paired zygomatic, partoid (near the ear), and mandibular glands are more distinct than the lobulated, spread-out sublingual glands. Salivary ducts transport the saliva from the glands to the duct openings in the oral cavity (upper fourth premolar, sublingual, etc.). Cats also have lingual and buccal molar glands.

Tonsils

Tonsils are typically situated in tonsillar crypts within the pharyngeal area. As lymphatic tissue, they can be reactive to conditions in the oral cavity, draining that region.

DENTAL ANATOMY

Knowing the proper terminology for dental structures will help you describe aberrations and assist you in communicating with others about your patients' oral conditions.

Terminology

The following distinctive terms are used in dentistry to identify structures and regions of the oral cavity (see Figure 1.2):

- *Mesial*: toward the front midline
- *Distal*: away from the front midline
- *Apical*: toward the apex (root)
- *Coronal*: toward the crown
- *Palatal*: toward the palate
- *Lingual*: toward the tongue
- *Buccal*: toward the cheek
- *Labial*: toward the lips
- *Facial*: labial or buccal
- *Occlusal*: facing a tooth in the opposite jaw
- *Interproximal*: surface between two teeth

Tooth Substance

The different layers of teeth are formed by the differentiation of cell lines to provide structures that function in mastication, defense, and grooming. Although there are differences among species as to shape and formation, the basic substances of teeth are common to all.

Figure 1.2 *Directional terminology*

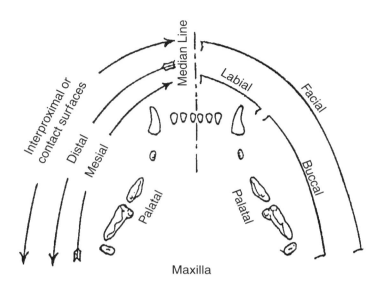

Maxilla

Mandible

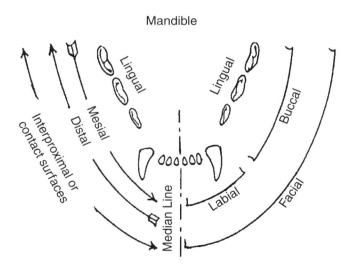

(Illustration adapted from original drawing by R. B. Wiggs)

Enamel

Enamel, covering the *crown* of the tooth, is the hardest and densest structure in the body, with a composition of 96% inorganic, primarily hydroxyapatite, crystals. Formed by *ameloblasts,* enamel has no regenerative capabilities once damaged.

Cementum

Cementum, covering the root of the tooth, is less dense than enamel (45 to 50% inorganic) and is secreted by *cementoblasts* during development. Cementoblasts that remain on the surface and cementocytes that become trapped in cellular cementum give the cementum the ability to regenerate. The cementoblasts also deposit cementum to hold the ends of the *periodontal membrane,* or *periodontal ligament* (PDL), in place (*Sharpey's fibers*).

Dentin

Dentin is found underneath the surface of both the enamel (in the crown) and the cementum (in the root). *Dentinal tubules* are formed by *odontoblasts,* and peritubular dentin makes up the bulk of the structure, with a 70% inorganic content. Odontoblastic processes "run up" the dentinal tubules, so if exposed, they can register pain or discomfort.

The odontoblasts continue to manufacture dentin throughout the life of the tooth, as demonstrated most vividly in the deposition of dentin that alters the wide canal of a young animal into a tooth that develops thicker dentinal walls and a thinner root canal as the animal ages. *Reparative dentin* can also be made to protect areas of dentinal loss or exposure.

Tooth Anatomy

The exposed part of the tooth seen above the gumline is the crown, and it is covered by enamel (see Figure 1.3). The root, or subgingival portion, is covered by cementum, and the two sections (crown and root) meet at the *neck* of the tooth, or the *cervical* region. Dentin underlies the enamel and cementum, in both the crown and the root of the tooth. The tip of the root is called the *apex.* Because dog and cat teeth complete normal growth when the apexes are closed (normally with no further *eruption*) and because their crowns are relatively short in comparison to their roots, these teeth are called *brachyodont* teeth.

Teeth may have one or more roots (normally up to three in dogs and cats). The space between the roots in multirooted teeth is called the *furcation.* If this region is ever exposed by loss of attachment (to the gingiva and bone) caused by periodontal disease, it is a difficult area to maintain properly.

Pulp Anatomy

The inner region of the *pulp cavity* will closely approximate the external anatomical form (see Figure 1.3). That part of the pulp cavity in the root is called the *root canal,* and the cavity in the crown is the *pulp chamber,* which has *pulpal horns* extending into the *cusps* of the crown.

In most domestic pets, the *pulp* vessels and nerves enter the tooth through an *apical delta.* This provides more of an apical stop or shelf than an apical foramen would (as seen in humans). The nerves can be stimulated by heat, cold, and pressure, but the sensation "felt" by the patient is pain.

Dental Formulas

The dog and cat both have two sets of teeth (diphyodont)—*deciduous* (temporary) and *permanent.* They typically have a specific number of teeth that erupt according to a generally predictable eruption timetable (see Table 1.1). The four types of teeth typically encountered are the incisors (I), canines, or *cuspids,* (C), premolars (P), and molars (M). A permanent tooth is often designated with a capital letter, and a deciduous tooth may be designated with a lowercase letter or by adding a "d" to the tooth letter. A tooth is often identified by placing its number (1, 2, 3 for first, second, third incisors; 1 for canines; 1, 2, 3, 4 for premolars; or 1, 2, 3 for molars) beside its letter type (I, C, P, or M) in the appropriate corner, as a superscript or subscript (referring to the animal's right or left side and upper or lower jaw, not as viewed). So, the upper right

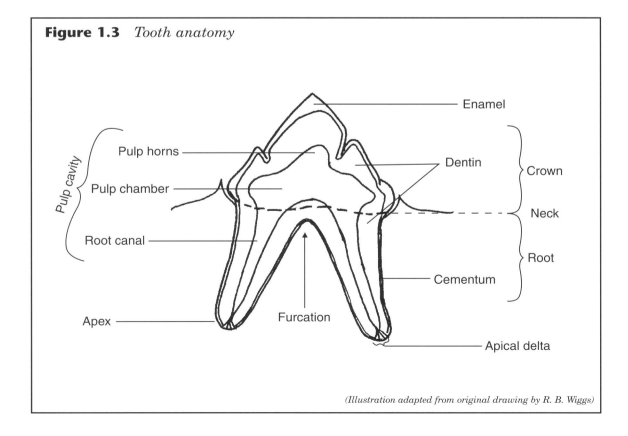

Figure 1.3 *Tooth anatomy*

(Illustration adapted from original drawing by R. B. Wiggs)

Table 1.1
Eruption times of teeth

	Deciduous teeth (weeks)	Permanent teeth (months)
Dogs		
Incisors	3–4	3–5
Canines	3	4–6
Premolars	4–12	4–6
Molars		5–7
Cats		
Incisors	2–3	3–4
Canines	3–4	4–5
Premolars	3–6	4–6
Molars		4–5

fourth premolar would be designated P^4, and the deciduous lower left third incisor would be $_3$Id. Another method of identification is known as the Triadan system. This system assigns a three-digit number to each tooth, with the first number denoting the quadrant and the last two digits specifying the tooth number. The quadrants are numbered from upper right (100) to upper left (200) to lower left (300) to lower right (400), and the teeth are numbered from the central incisor back (incisors 01, 02, 03; canines 04; premolars 05 to 08; molars 09 to 11). Thus, the upper right fourth premolar would be 108, and the deciduous lower left third incisor would be 703 (deciduous teeth range from the 500s to the 800s).

Feline dental formulas are as follows:

> Deciduous: $2 \times$ (Id 3/3; Cd 1/1; Pd 3/2) = 26 teeth
> Permanent: $2 \times$ (I 3/3; C 1/1; P 3/2; M 1/1) = 30 teeth

Note that the cat's permanent premolars are numbered 2, 3, and 4 in the maxilla and 3 and 4 in the mandible.

Similarly, canine dental formulas are as follows:

> Deciduous: $2 \times$ (Id 3/3; Cd 1/1; Pd 3/3) = 28 teeth
> Permanent: $2 \times$ (I 3/3; C 1/1; P 4/4; M 3/2) = 42 teeth

ERUPTION TIMES

Exact eruption times need not be memorized, but it is important to know that there should not be two teeth of the same type in the same place at the same time (i.e., there should be no *retained* or *persistent deciduous teeth*). When such an event occurs, the deciduous teeth must be carefully extracted.

Great care should always be taken when dealing with deciduous teeth because even at a younger age (6 to 8 weeks), the permanent tooth buds are just below the surface of the deciduous teeth, and any traumatic elevation could damage the permanent bud.

Proper Occlusion

To get the most comfortable and functional bite, an animal's occlusion should be in proper relation. The following relationships between teeth can be evaluated for occlusion:

- Upper incisors in front of lower incisors (scissor-incisor bite relation)
- Lower canine teeth fitting evenly between the upper canine and third incisor (not tight against the incisor)
- Premolars in a "pinking-shear" configuration (the tips of the cusps of the mandibular premolars pointing directly into the interdigital spaces of the maxillary premolars, with the cusps overlapping in a horizontal plane)
- Cusps of the upper fourth premolars being lateral (buccal) to the lower first molars

Specific abnormalities and *malocclusions* will be discussed in chapter 5: Advanced Oral and Dental Problems.

Periodontium

The structures around the tooth that support it—known as the *periodontium*—are extremely important, for they keep the tooth in the osseous structure of the head. These structures include the cementum of the root, the periodontal ligament, the alveolus, and the *gingiva*. The cementum, as discussed earlier, remains vital with cementoblasts producing cementum, which helps in connecting the ends of the periodontal ligament (Sharpey's fibers) to the tooth.

The periodontal ligament is primarily composed of collagen from fibroblasts and has many different types of fibers, categorized according to where they are found and what they connect. Most of the fibers run between the alveolus (described previously), or alveolar socket, with Sharpey's fibers of the PDL embedded in the alveolar bone and the remainder of the ligament extending to the cementum of the tooth. Additional fibers may also run from the gingiva to the alveolar bone or tooth, around the tooth, or between adjacent teeth. In addition to helping support the tooth within the alveolus, the periodontal ligament protects underlying tissue from bacterial invasion, provides a "shock-absorbing" system, and is even responsible for some of the sensations a tooth may experience.

Covering this underlying supporting tissue, the *attached gingiva* is the mouth's first line of defense against bacteria in the oral cavity. The attached gingiva is that portion of the gum tissue closest to the crown of the tooth. It is often demarcated by the *mucogingival line* (or *mucogingival junction*) from the looser buccal mucosa "below" it. The attached gingiva is even histologically different from the rest of the *oral mucosa* because of the additional connective tissue (rete pegs) that keep it tightly adhered to the underlying bone. A minimum of 2 to 3 mm of attached gingiva is necessary to protect underlying tissues. The edge of the gingiva itself is often not directly attached to the tooth for a short distance and is called the *free gingiva* or *free gingival margin*. The space between the free gingival margin and tooth is called the *gingival sulcus,* and at the depth of the sulcus is the *junctional epithelium,* or the site of attachment to the tooth typically at the neck or *cementoenamel* junction. In a normal dog, a sulcus depth may be 1 to 3 mm in depth, but in a cat, a sulcus depth of barely 0.5 mm is typically seen.

CHAPTER 2

Oral Examination and Recognition of Pathology

ORAL EXAMINATION

As in every other discipline in veterinary medicine, a practitioner must use a combination of knowledge and observation in dentistry, comparing abnormal findings with known normals, to determine the best course of action. It is imperative that every patient possible have a thorough oral exam, not only to permit the practitioner to become familiar with normal expectations, including breed variations, but also, of course, to detect pathology.

History

Veterinary professionals often have to rely on information provided by astute owners who relate their pets' ongoing symptoms, such as difficulty in eating or swallowing, excess salivation, swelling, drainage, oral odor, or indications of oral pain or discomfort. This information, coupled with a complete history (including past oral problems and treatments, as well as vaccination and viral status, diet, chewing behavior, and home care), can give a more complete picture of influences on the oral cavity. Many systemic events affect the oral cavity, and the rest of the body can, in turn, be affected by oral disease, so the patient and its history must be thoroughly examined.

External Examination

It is a good idea to gather initial information while observing the patient's body overall, instead of going abruptly to an oral examination. Everything from body condition (thinness, unkempt coat) to the symmetry of the facial structures should be noted during a gradual "introduction" to the patient. Special attention should be paid to areas of swelling or even drainage that might be associated with the oral cavity. There are, however, some patients who will allow no more than an arm's-length assessment without some form of sedation!

Initial Oral Examination (Alert Patient)

If the patient is amenable to further observation, an initial oral assessment on the exam table can give you a preliminary insight into what oral and dental disease may be present. Movements around the head should be quiet and gentle, as some patients are head-shy even when completely healthy, and those in pain may become agitated with forced manipulation. Depending on the patient, a wide range of procedures may be accomplished, from a simple observation of tooth surfaces (noting *calculus* present, broken teeth, gingival inflammation, etc.) to a probing of open canals and pocket depths. The oral soft tissues should also be evaluated, including the sublingual area, by pressing a finger up into the submandibular space when opening the mouth. Palatal and pharyngeal inflammation and foreign bodies may be noticed, and any abnormalities in the tonsillar size and appearance should be noted.

Complete Oral Examination (Patient under Anesthesia or Sedation)

Although some patients might allow a great deal of examination while they are awake, it is impossible to get a full assessment without some form of sedation, usually general anesthesia. In addition, most dental procedures cannot and should not be performed without full anesthesia and a cuffed endotracheal tube in place. Proper preanesthetic assessment of total body condition and function, with proper monitoring and support, will reduce the chance of complications. Though not completely free of risk, the newer anesthetic products have greatly enhanced the ability to provide quality dental services while minimizing the risk to the patient.

Once the patient is completely under anesthesia, with a cuffed endotracheal tube in place, a thorough dental and oral evaluation can be performed. Good visibility enhanced by proper lighting, adequate mouth props, and even magnification greatly improves your ability to fully observe the oral cavity. Many tools can be used in the evaluation, including a periodontal explorer-probe, mirrors, lighting, and even radiology. A systematic method of recording any abnormalities is essential in order to develop accurate medical records, to avoid overlooking areas, and to be able to discuss any conditions encountered with other individuals, including the owner. Many types of dental records may be used, including stickers or stamps for records or separate dental record sheets. The following sections offer a brief outline of conditions to assess in the oral structures.

Teeth

The teeth should be evaluated for number (too few, too many), shape (microdontia, macrodontia), structure (fractures, pitted enamel), color (*pulpitis,* tetracycline deposition), position (rotation, malocclusion), stability (mobility present), and materials on the surface (*plaque* and calculus).

Gingiva

The oral soft tissue should be assessed for color variation (icteric, cyanotic, pale, hemorrhagic), swelling (ulceration, edema, tumor, hyperplasia), attachment (loss of tissue), and topography. In addition, an important indicator of periodontal disease is the extent of the gingival sulcus or pocket in relation to the level of attachment of the periodontium. This will be covered in more detail in chapter 3: Periodontal Disease.

Osseous Structures

The palpation of hard tissues is often best accompanied by radiographs to detect any loss of integrity, including periodontal bone loss, traumatic injury (fractures, *avulsions*), and even the articulation of the temporomandibular joint (TMJ). Osseous assessment can also play a role in occlusal evaluation if the jaw size relationship is abnormal.

METHODS OF EXAMINATION

A thorough examination makes use of and integrates several different means and tools to gather information. The most important method you can implement is oral radiography, which is an integral part of veterinary dentistry.

Visual

Astute observation is the practitioner's initial means of trying to locate abnormalities, particularly when dealing with changes of color and structure. In the oral cavity, the olfactory sense may be bombarded as well!

Tactile

No oral exam is complete without a physical assessment of the oral tissues, particularly those of the periodontium. Accurate diagnosis and treatment planning is impossible without some form of gingival pocket depth evaluation, and a *periodontal probe* is made for just that purpose (see chapter 9: Materials and Equipment) (Figure 2.1). Ideally, each tooth should be gently probed at six sites around the tooth, and care should always be taken to avoid pushing the probe tip through the junctional epithelium

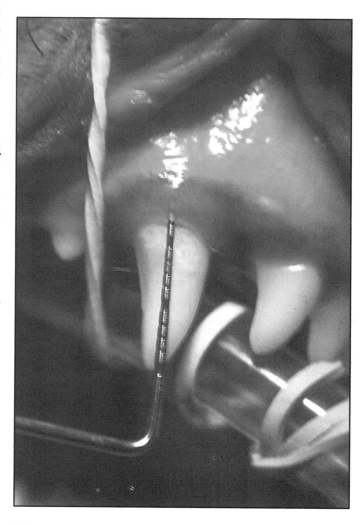

Figure 2.1 *Periodontal probe in sulcus*

at the depth of the pocket, particularly if the tissues are inflamed and therefore more fragile.

Most periodontal probes have a periodontal explorer on the opposite end. This thin, sharp-tipped end is an extremely tactile instrument and can be used (carefully) to detect hidden calculus in pocket depths. At times, the explorer is also useful in trying to determine if there has been canal exposure resulting from a crown fracture or *attrition,* as the narrow tip of the instrument often fits into the canal opening. The sharp explorer tip will "stick" in soft, carious enamel or catch on the rough edge of a resorptive lesion. The twitch response from the patient, even under full anesthesia, is often a telltale sign as well.

Temperature

Assessing sensitivity to temperature differentials is often quite helpful in diagnosing the extent of pulpal involvement in humans, but getting a consistent response from an alert veterinary patient is another matter. Using water frozen in a tuberculin syringe to watch for cold sensitivity is an option, but accurate communication of specific areas of discomfort can be very subjective. Heat sensitivity, though an indicator of potentially more serious problems, is even more difficult to assess.

Transillumination

Using a focused light source behind a tooth (*transillumination*) often helps determine tooth vitality, with a nonvital tooth not allowing light to filter through as well as a vital tooth. Although interpreting the findings is a fairly subjective business, coupling this technique with a full exam and oral radiographs can help give a complete picture of the situation.

Radiography

No matter how thorough a visual examination is, there can always be underlying changes that only radiography can reveal. For example, it is virtually impossible to determine the extent of periodontal attachment loss, the involvement of root *resorption* in erosive lesions in cats, or *periapical* lesions, among others, without the use of radiographs.

Extraoral Radiographs

Although some good survey films may help you obtain an adequate overall picture in cases involving head trauma, tumors, general bone density, or malformations, extraoral radiographs generally are not sufficient to allow the localization of a specific area of the oral cavity. No matter how good the technique of oblique views is, there is nearly always some additional structure superimposed over the area in question.

Intraoral Radiographs

By using a radiographic film inside the oral cavity, you can eliminate most of the problems encountered with the superimposition of other structures. A standard cassette can be used in a larger animal by placing the corner of the cassette in the mouth; smaller dental intraoral films, with their convenience and flexibility, are invaluable.

The most common size of intraoral film used in veterinary dentistry is probably size 2 film (1½ in. × 1⁹⁄₁₆ in.) (Figure 2.2). Sizes 0 and 1 (which are both smaller) and size 2 are considered periapical films, as the focus for their images is typically the root structure. Size 4 film (2¼ in. × 3 in.), or occlusal film, is often used in the rostral portion of the oral cavity to visualize the incisors and canines. This size of film is also extremely helpful in taking whole-body radiographs of small birds and rodents and even in X-raying the extremities of small dogs and cats. Size 3 films are longer than size 2 films but of similar width, and they have a bitewing tab, which facilitates their use in human dentistry to view the crowns of upper and lower teeth. In animals, these films allow a view of more teeth in dogs with longer arches. Film speeds D and E are the most common types used currently.

Because these small films are double-emulsion, nonscreen films, you can get good detail on radiographs at a reasonable price. The film is often encased in a layer of black paper, with a lead sheet on the "back" side to prevent back scatter when the film is exposed (Figure 2.3). These materials are enclosed in a plastic or water-resistant, "light-tight" cover for additional protection. An embossed *"dimple,"* often palpable through all layers, is used for properly orienting the film in the mouth.

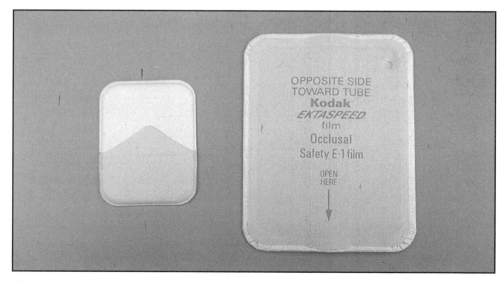

Figure 2.2 *Size 2 (periapical) and size 4 (occlusal) intraoral films, with embossed dimple visible on upper right corner of size 4 film*

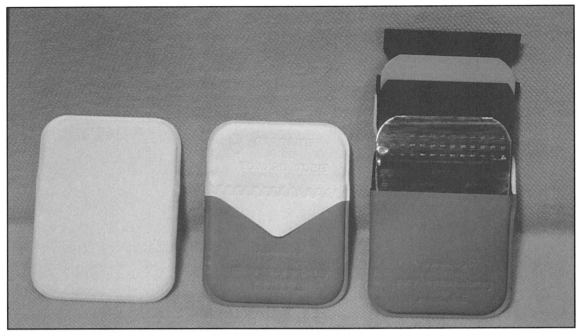

Figure 2.3 *Intraoral film packet, opened to show components*

The film itself is placed in the oral cavity with the white side, "dimple," or convexity facing toward the radiographic source. The words "opposite side toward tube" are often printed on the back to avoid confusion (Figure 2.2). If the film is placed upside down, the X rays will pass through the lead sheet first, and the image will show the stippling of the imprinted pattern on the lead sheet and be underexposed. Consistently having the dimple toward the X-ray source will help in identifying the structures in the images.

Radiographic Technique

The size and flexibility of the intraoral films make them very convenient, but you must learn a level of technique sensitivity to become proficient in dental radiography. Ideally, you would have access to a dental radiographic unit, but in most clinics, the standard radiographic unit can be used with a little practice.

Standard Radiographic Unit Technique. A mobile radiographic head offers some advantages in taking intraoral films, but it is not a necessity. Being able to lower the standard unit head shortens the focal distance, thereby decreasing the amount of distortion and reducing the exposure time. The ideal focal distance is around 12 inches from the film, which, in many cases, places the unit very close to the patient's head. With a milliampere (mA) setting of 100, the time can be set to $\frac{1}{16}$ to $\frac{1}{10}$ of a second at a focal distance of 12 inches or $\frac{2}{5}$ to $\frac{3}{5}$ of a second at a stationary focal distance of 36 to 42 inches. Because each unit is unique, it is helpful to make a technique chart for the unit you will be using, with specimens of different sizes. Generally, a guideline of 65 kVp for a small dog or cat and up to 85 kVp for a giant breed is a good place to start. The ability to rotate the X-ray head has benefits in positioning, which will be discussed.

Film Placement. The typical approach of placing a film close to the object being examined, with the object and film relatively parallel to each other and the primary beam aimed perpendicular to both, is called the *parallel technique* (Figure 2.4). Although this method can be used in many other areas of the body and with limbs, only one area of the oral cavity is amenable to such a technique—the area of the mandibular premolars and molars. In this method, the intraoral film is placed to the inside of the teeth and gently introduced down into the intermandibular space, and the beam is aimed directly toward the teeth. If necessary, the patient's head can be adjusted to position the film so that it is parallel to the table as well.

In all other areas of the oral cavity, however, it is very difficult to place the film parallel to the tooth and root. To minimize distortion and to obtain an image that is similar in size and form to the object being examined, a

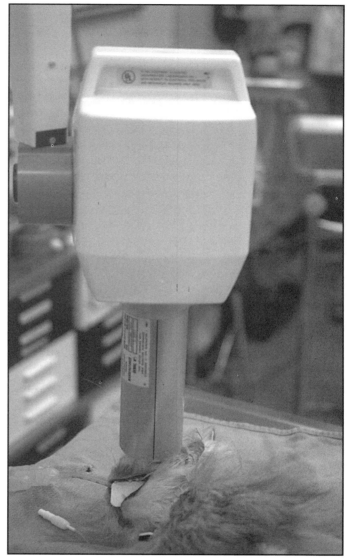

Figure 2.4 *Intraoral parallel technique, feline mandible*

method called the *bisecting angle technique* (Figure 2.5) must be utilized. The premise behind such a technique takes into consideration the fact that the film and the object actually diverge from each other, like two sides of an angle. If the beam were aimed perpendicular to the tooth, the image would be elongated on the film, and if the beam were aimed perpendicular to the film, the image would be foreshortened. Therefore, by aiming the beam perpendicular to a line that lies between the two (the film and the long axis of the tooth or root), a

Figure 2.5 *Bisecting angle technique*

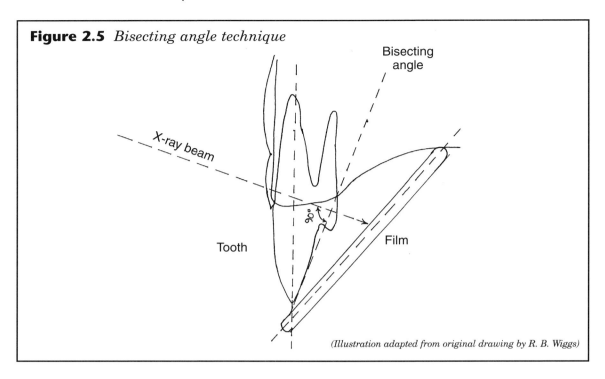

(Illustration adapted from original drawing by R. B. Wiggs)

Figure 2.6 *Patient's head positioned for bisecting angle technique*

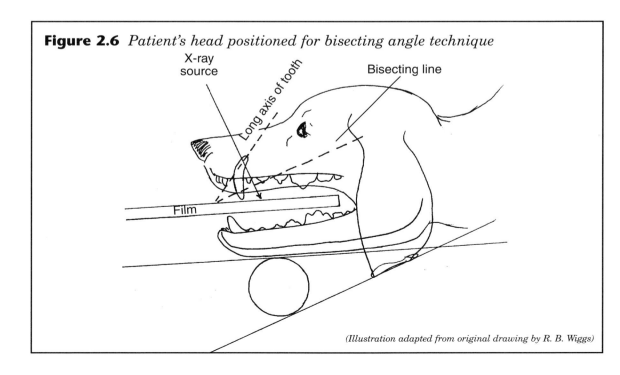

(Illustration adapted from original drawing by R. B. Wiggs)

compromise results in an image that is similar in size to the object, though some distortion will still be present.

With a radiographic head that is mobile (or a dental X-ray unit), the X-ray source can be rotated until the beam is directed perpendicular to this bisecting line. If stationary, the patient's head must then be positioned so that the bisecting line is parallel to the table and therefore perpendicular to the beam (Figure 2.6). This seems confusing in print, and it sometimes takes a bit of practice to get the technique down, but by using different aids (such as a penlight or three dowels, swabs, or sticks connected together to approximate the angle and line), adequate films aren't too difficult to attain. Moreover, the technique is well worth learning given the detail and isolation of the area that can be achieved when performed correctly. Intraoral films are relatively inexpensive, so it is feasible to practice on a skull not only to enhance your ability in positioning but also to work out a technique chart showing the kilovolt peak for the particular machine you'll be using.

Developing Films

Developing intraoral films offers a range of options as well. Again, you can use what you have on hand. If you use standard tanks and solutions, you can either grasp the small film with a pair of hemostats (or purchase intraoral film clips) or keep the solutions in smaller containers in the darkroom: Once a small film is lost at the bottom of a large tank, it's gone forever. This method will take just as long as developing and fixing a regular film, with variables of temperature and "age" of solutions.

An automatic processor can also be used. The intraoral film can be taped to the lead edge of a regular sheet of X-ray film, but the amount of solutions used will be wasted on the unused portion of the leader film, and the tape can obscure part of the small film's image. Some companies make specific carriers for intraoral film use in automatic processors.

Ideally, rapid dental developers and fixers can be used in a *chairside developer* placed beside the dental table in the operatory (Figure 2.7). With fresh solutions, films can be ready to read in less than a minute—without requiring you to leave the patient's side. These solutions can also be placed in small containers in the darkroom to get faster developing and fixing times, but the convenience of a chairside developer is enormous. Ultimately, the more convenient and "comfortable" intraoral radiography becomes, the more likely it is to be used, benefiting both the patients and the clinic's bottom line!

Reading Films: Interpretation

Once the film is developed, a systematic regimen for reading the films should be followed. Use the dimple that is embossed on the film to help you orient the film's position and identify the teeth imaged. Though the method employed varies from clinic to clinic, we typically hold the film and look "into" the dimple, envisioning that we are looking at the lingual surface of the teeth (as if standing on the tongue, looking out). From there and by knowing basic anatomy, we can determine if we are looking at the upper or lower jaw, and we can adjust the film according to sequential tooth order (incisors to canines to

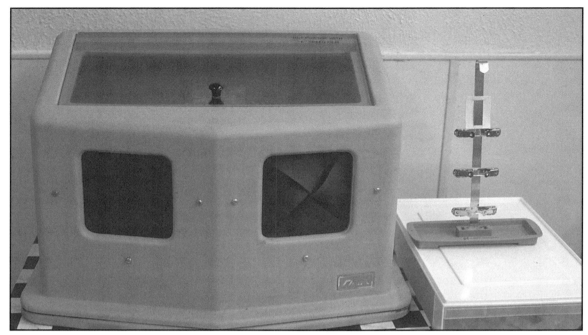

Figure 2.7a *Chairside developer for intraoral films*

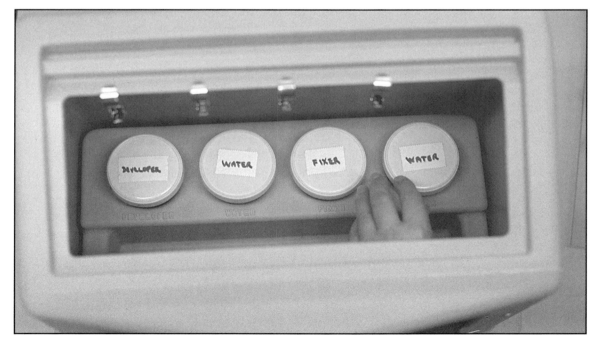

Figure 2.7b *Inside view of chairside developer with plastic safety cover removed*

premolars to molars), which then tells us if the image is of the right or left side. The alternate method of looking at the films with the dimple out (toward you) is preferred by some and considered to be more consistent with a buccal view (as if looking from outside the mouth).

Normal Anatomy. Only by reading many films can you become acquainted with what is considered normal anatomy and therefore be able to recognize what is abnormal (Figure 2.8). Entire texts have been written on oral radiology, but we'll cover some basic points here. Optimally, in a normal anatomy, the entire tooth structure, including the root and apex, is visible. There is no evidence of fracture or damage to the tooth (it should have a smooth outer contour), and the tooth is well seated into the alveolus. The periodontal ligament space is recognized as the radiolucent space between the tooth and the denser lamina dura, the cortical plate of the alveolus. Although certain osseous structures may help identify structures (such as the *incisive foramen* of the maxillae and the *mandibular symphysis*), others may mimic pathology, such as the radiolucent mandibular foramina or even the opening of the infraorbital canal.

The tooth anatomy itself can be assessed, from the enamel covering the crown to the root structure. The thickness of the dentinal wall underneath the enamel and cementum gives clues to the age of the patient or of the tooth. Young animals, for example, have very thin dentinal walls and wide-open canals, at times visible radiographically in a blunderbuss configuration, often

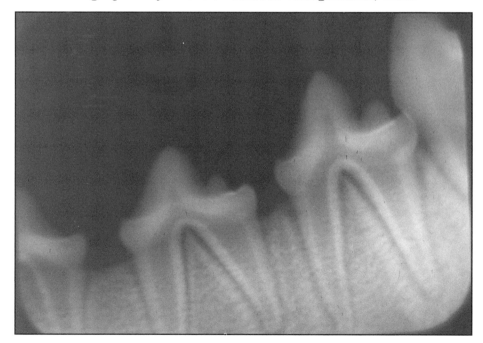

Figure 2.8 *Normal radiographic anatomy of the mandible of a young dog; periodontal ligament space seen as radiolucent line between the root and the radiopaque lamina dura of the alveolar bone*

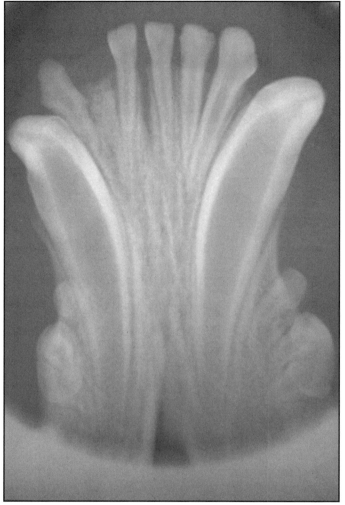

Figure 2.9 *Immature mandibular canines, with wider canal and open apexes*

with the apex not fully closed (Figure 2.9). As the animal matures, dentin is deposited toward the center of the tooth and pulp space, and the space narrows. Similarly, to determine if a tooth is still vital, you can compare the size of its canal to that of similar teeth. A tooth with a wider canal has probably been nonvital for some time and should be treated accordingly.

Radiographs are also helpful in determining if permanent tooth buds are present in a young dog who still has all its deciduous teeth. Such images will reveal the close proximity of the developing permanent tooth buds to the deciduous tooth roots. This is extremely important to keep in mind when working with any deciduous teeth, especially when extracting them, because it does not take much to traumatize the sensitive buds.

Bone Loss. Probably the most common reason to take intraoral radiographs is to assess the bone structure surrounding the teeth—not just the teeth themselves. Certainly, in periodontal disease (see chapter 3: Periodontal Disease), radiographs are a vital tool in assessing the amount of attachment loss, particularly bone loss. Crestal bone loss occurs earliest, and varying patterns of bone loss may determine how successful therapy will be. Vertical bone loss occurs down the roots of a tooth, often with significant pocket depths, and it is sometimes amenable to some form of regenerative periodontal therapy. Horizontal bone loss is a more even loss across multiple teeth (Figure 2.10), and pockets may not be a problem if gingival *recession* has also occurred, but root and furcation exposure would require treatment or monitoring or both.

Bone loss can also occur as a result of the endodontic compromise of the pulp. Once a pulp is injured or becomes nonvital, it can become infected, either

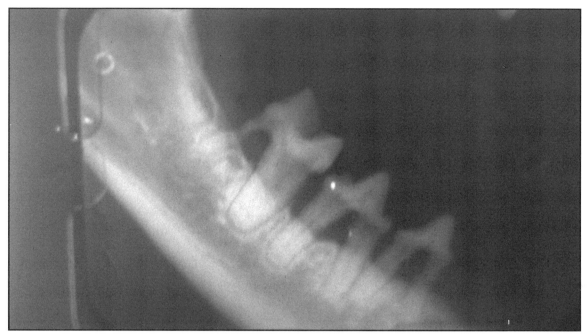

Figure 2.10 *Horizontal bone loss (feline mandible)*

through the exposure site or anachoretically. Once infected, the bacteria goes into the periapical region, and a *periapical abscess* or granuloma can result, often represented by a radiolucent halo around the apex of the root (Figure 2.11). Once the pulp and periapical tissues are involved, some means of therapy must be undertaken to remove the source of infection—either extraction or endodontics to clean the pulp space and seal it. Radiography is especially important in those cases that do not seem serious (tooth fracture, canal apparently not open) but that may have hidden problems.

    Resorptive Lesions. Radiographs are also a "must" for any level of treatment of resorptive lesions in cats (see chapter 7: Feline Oral and Dental Disease). When you consider filling a tooth that has only a shallow lesion, a radiograph must be taken because, even in such a tooth, there may well be involvement of the roots, with internal resorption, external resorption, or both. If extraction is selected (as it should be in the great majority of cases), a preoperative film will show you how involved the roots are. If the roots are reasonably intact and the periodontal ligament (PDL) is visible, the proper steps of extraction should be followed, just as they would be in any other situation. Complications come with those roots in which resorption has already started and bone is already "growing into" the teeth. Complete extraction may be difficult with these teeth, and care must be taken to avoid excessive injury to the jaw during extraction and pulverization techniques.

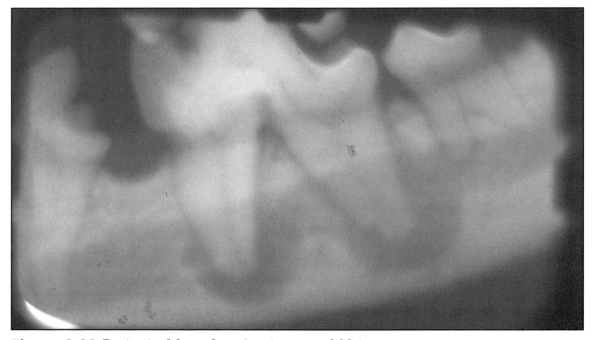

Figure 2.11 *Periapical bone loss (canine mandible)*

Neoplasia. Survey extraoral films may be taken initially to determine the overall involvement of oral neoplasia in the hard tissues, but intraoral films will allow you to localize a specific area. Thus, you can more accurately assess the extent of the lesion and therefore plan appropriate therapy. If resection is the chosen treatment, postoperative radiographs of both the operative site and the removed section can aid in evaluation.

COMMON ORAL AND DENTAL PATHOLOGY

Although some lesions in the oral cavity may be fairly obvious, only by systematically looking through the region will a thorough assessment be possible. The recognition of abnormalities integrates a knowledge of normal anatomy and physiology with an understanding of how aberrations can affect the patient as a whole.

Periodontal Disease

Recognized as the most common infectious disease in man and pets, periodontal disease is by far the most frequently seen oral problem. As such, it will be discussed in greater detail in chapter 3: Periodontal Disease.

Dental Abnormalities

Abnormalities in tooth number (*supernumerary teeth,* or extra teeth; *oligodontia,* or some missing teeth; *anodontia,* or no teeth), shape (extra roots, microdontia, macrodontia), and roots (*fusion tooth,* supernumerary) are not uncommon in pets. Often, such variations are incidental findings without significant problems, unless crowding from extra teeth predisposes the patient to periodontal disease.

Additional variations, such as the fusion of two teeth, gemination (attempted incomplete "twinning"), and more extensive formation abnormalities (for example, *dens-in-dente* with potential pulp exposure), may be found. If the integrity of the pulp chamber is compromised, the tooth must be adequately treated.

Variations in the eruption sequence can range from a delayed eruption schedule to retained deciduous teeth to submerged teeth. All sites with "missing" teeth should always be radiographed because if the permanent tooth is unerupted, developmental cells around the neck can cause extreme cystic development, which can damage surrounding bone (Figure 2.12). A *dentigerous cyst* is usually apparent as a radiographic halo around a submerged tooth and can be quite extensive. Another form of incomplete eruption may be present as an *operculum,* a thick, tough, fibrous coating of gingiva that appears to be obstructing further eruption. At times, the tooth can be almost fully erupted but still covered with the thick tissue. Excision to expose the tooth may allow further eruption if the tooth is still developing (open root).

Crown

Abnormalities of the crown are often seen, the result of causes ranging from genetic to acquired.

Enamel Hypocalcification and Hypoplasia. When pitting and discoloration of the enamel is seen in young pets (primarily dogs), using the term *enamel hypoplasia* for the condition is often not completely accurate. This condition typically is characterized by adequate enamel production, so it is not hypoplastic. However, mineralization has been insufficient because of an influence during formation, such as fever or inflammation (thus the term *distemper teeth*), resulting in *enamel hypocalcification.* This softer enamel is worn away more easily and is often discolored (Plate 1*). This condition may be generalized (a long-standing inflammation) or localized to specific teeth, sometimes even appearing in distinct bands, reflecting the finite period of time since the insult occurred. Any teeth with enamel changes should also be radiographed to monitor for root abnormalities.

Enamel Staining. The enamel can appear discolored either from substances within it or the underlying dentin (intrinsic—e.g., from tetracycline) or from materials on the enamel (extrinsic—e.g., materials picked up during metal chewing). Unless this type of color change is associated with some

---

* Plates are located mid-book, beginning on page 63.

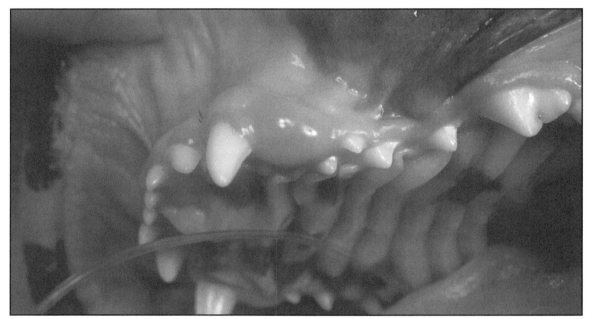

Figure 2.12a *Cystic structure (dentigerous cyst)*

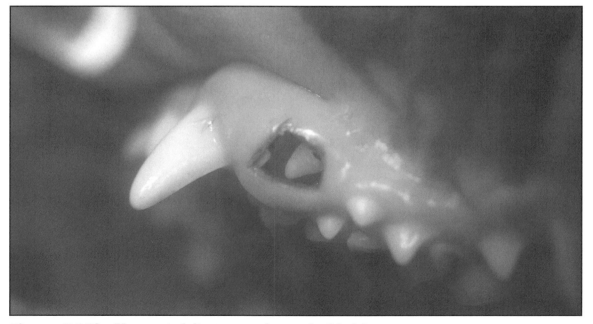

Figure 2.12b *Unerupted first premolar embedded in cyst*

pathology, such aspulpitis (see next paragraph) or excessive wear, the staining is often of little consequence (other than aesthetic considerations).

Pulpitis. When blunt trauma damages the pulp and causes hemorrhage, the crown will exhibit a pinkish tint from the bleeding into the dentinal tubules. If minor, such pulpitis may be reversible, and the color should revert to normal. If excessive damage has been done and the pulp is irreversibly damaged, however, the color will often change to darker hues such as purple or gray, and the degradation products of the red blood cells will accumulate in the tubules (Plate 2). Although there may be no external signs of damage to the tooth, such a structure must be considered nonvital and should be handled appropriately. Radiographs can help confirm a nonvital tooth or periapical bone loss.

Attrition. Chewing on abrasive objects can cause a significant loss of tooth enamel and dentin. If the wear, or *attrition,* is gradual enough, the odontoblasts continue to form a reparative dentin in the "roof" of the pulp chamber, thereby lowering its height to avoid exposure of the pulp. Such a tooth may have a dark-brown center (reparative dentin) but no distinct canal opening. In assessing the tooth, it is helpful to confirm the signs of tooth vitality by radiographs (a vital tooth will have a proper diameter in the canal and no periapical changes). A specific pattern of attrition may be seen in dogs who chew on the bars or chains of their cages. The loss of enamel and dentin on the distal surfaces of the canine teeth can be severe enough to expose the pulp and endanger the entire structure of the tooth.

Trauma. Traumatic forces to a tooth can result in a more rapid loss of tooth structure, which can acutely expose the pulp chamber and necessitate proper therapy. Some tooth fractures occur without pulp exposure, but they should be assessed radiographically and monitored in the future to ascertain continued pulp vitality.

Teeth can also be avulsed from the alveolus, either partially (luxated) or completely; at times, this process can also affect some of the surrounding bone. To plan the course of treatment, you should fully assess the integrity of the affected tissues and determine whether the pulpal blood supply has been interrupted.

Caries and Resorptive Lesions. Actual cavities, or carious lesions, can be found in pets, but they are not that common. Occasionally, lesions may be seen on the occlusive surfaces of the molars in dogs, exhibiting as anything from a spot of soft enamel to extensive structural tooth loss (Figure 2.13). Shallow lesions without extensive involvement can be restored, but extraction is often the only option.

Resorptive lesions, seen primarily in cats but sometimes in dogs, are not true carious lesions. Much is still to be determined about these lesions, but the fact that they are often progressive factors into the treatment choice. A more in-depth discussion can be found in chapter 7: Feline Oral and Dental Disease.

Roots

Abnormalities involving the roots often cannot be fully evaluated without the use of oral radiology. Obviously, no matter how good the crown looks, if the root is not stable the tooth will not stay in the alveolus.

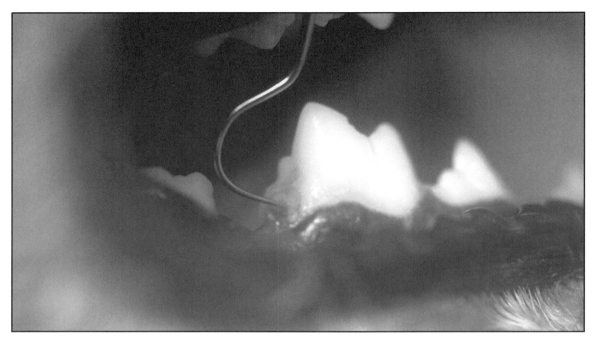

Figure 2.13a *Severe carious lesion of distal cusp of mandibular first molar*

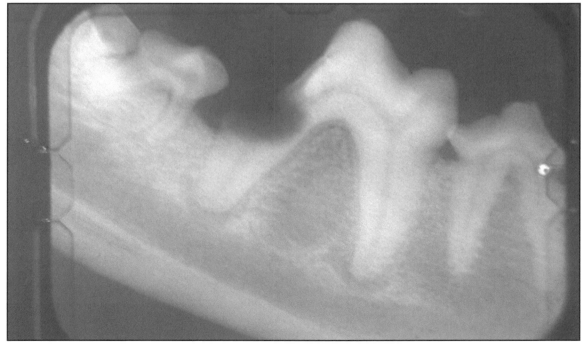

Figure 2.13b *Radiograph of carious lesion*

Resorption. Both internal and external resorption of the roots can be readily seen in many cases of feline resorptive lesions, as would be expected. Any inflammation in the pulp space itself can instigate an internal resorptive pattern with destruction of the dentinal walls. Often, more external forces (osteoclasts) will be involved with external resorption of the roots. Loss of clarity of the root outline will be seen radiographically.

Ankylosis. A level of resorption and certainly inflammation can lead to the obliteration of the periodontal ligament and space, causing the alveolar bone to fuse to the cementum. Masticatory forces, especially when excessive, can, over time, cause such changes. In feline resorptive lesions, ankylosis may be seen radiographically, particularly when the root becomes almost completely remodeled into bone.

Trauma. Even though they are encased in bone, roots are very susceptible to traumatic forces. Root-crown fractures are not uncommon, whether at a *fulcrum* point or a fracture line extending subgingivally. With few exceptions, the instability of such fractures can make treatment challenging.

Gingiva and Mucosa

Beyond the specific gingival abnormalities associated with periodontal disease, the oral soft tissues can reflect the current status of the mouth and of the entire body as well.

Gingival Hyperplasia

The boxer breed often comes to mind when thinking of gingival hyperplasia, and certainly there is a familial predisposition to this condition in these dogs. Although the hyperplasia is actually a benign overgrowth of the attached gingiva (often generalized), it can be quite extensive, in some cases even covering sections of teeth. The increase in gingival height leads to the formation of deep "pseudopockets" that have significant pocket depths yet maintain proper attachment-level height. Reduction of the excessive tissue to reduce the pockets and better expose the teeth is often recommended.

Tumors and Masses

The oral cavity may be the site of various types of abnormal masses, including malignant tumors, which will be discussed at the end of this chapter. Any suspicious lesion should be biopsied.

Epulides. These tumors have been classified in different ways, but the general aspects of epulides are the same. They arise from the periodontal ligament, so therapy should include removal of the PDL, with extraction as a necessary adjunct. The fibrous and ossifying epulides contain components described by their names (fibrous tissue, ossified tissue). Depending on the involvement of the underlying bone, extraction and curettage may suffice for treatment.

Of the three basic forms of epulides, the *acanthomatous epulis* is by far the most aggressive, often affecting sizable regions of the mandible or maxilla, yet it is still considered benign. Such tumors will require wider margins of excision, and recurrence is often likely (Plate 3). Radiographs are very helpful in assessing location.

Systemic Disease

Just as the eyes can reflect many diseases, so can the oral cavity lead the practitioner to a discovery of systemic problems. Conditions such as anemia, icterus, and cyanosis are often assessed by gingival color. Bleeding disorders with petechia are sometimes first noticed in the oral cavity, as are autoimmune diseases with ulcerative mucosal surfaces.

Trauma

Hard oral tissues (teeth, bone) are often focused upon after a traumatic episode, but the soft tissues should also be closely evaluated for any injuries. Sutured gingival tears can help protect underlying tissues, particularly bone. Care should always be taken to try to preserve adequate amounts of attached gingiva.

"Gum-Chewer's Syndrome." Self-inflicted trauma as a result of the pet chewing on the inside of the cheek or even the tongue can cause a proliferative, granulomatous hyperplasia to occur. If the chewing is mild, only minimal signs of damage are seen; in serious cases, however, large chunks of tissue can be chewed on to the point of regular hemorrhage, and they can become painful.

Tongue

All surfaces of the tongue should be observed and even palpated. Sublingual tissues should also be examined for abnormalities or foreign bodies.

Inflammation

Glossitis may be present for a number of reasons—viral, immune-mediated (autoimmune, lymphocytic-plasmacytic *stomatitis*), or toxic—as well as exposure to irritative substances or objects. Uremia may result in ulceration of the tongue and oral tissues. Lesions of unknown origin should be biopsied for further diagnostic workup. In addition, it is sometimes helpful to correlate lingual lesions to other abnormalities in the oral cavity.

Trauma

Because many pets use their tongues to explore and taste new objects, traumatic lingual lesions can occur in these structures. Small lacerations, particularly under the tongue, can be quite sensitive and affect an animal's ability to eat properly. Foreign objects, especially strings, can get caught around the base of the tongue, potentially causing severe problems if they extend into the intestinal tract. Mechanical irritation from licking harsh or abrasive objects can cause significant ulceration and even granuloma formation if the material becomes embedded in the tongue. One case of nearly complete lingual avulsion was resolved satisfactorily when the dog learned how to prehend food and water with a much shorter tongue. Cats, however, do not fare as well with portions of the tongue missing, particularly in eating and grooming.

Developmental Abnormalities

Tongues can be larger than normal (macroglossia) or have a firm connection to sublingual tissue (a "tongue-tied" condition). A more serious condition can sometimes be found in newborn puppies when the tongue fails to develop normally. A puppy with *"bird tongue,"* a narrow tongue, is unable to nurse properly and often dies young, sometimes being underdiagnosed with the catchall phrase "fading puppy syndrome." Puppies with this condition who are force-fed have shown severe abnormalities in many other body systems, so support and therapy is not recommended.

Neoplasia

The tongue and sublingual tissues are among the more common sites for squamous cell carcinoma (SCC) in the cat. Other tumors are possible (melanoma, etc.) but are not common. Eosinophilic plaques can be found, and biopsy is the only sure way to get an accurate diagnosis.

Osseous Tissues

Lesions of the bones of the oral cavity can sometimes be handled improperly if standard techniques for treating long bones are used. Although stabilization of the bones is always important, occlusion must be maintained in the oral cavity.

Developmental Abnormalities

In some young terriers, including West Highland white, Scottish, and Cairn terriers, a bilateral swelling of the mandibles may occur. This *craniomandibular osteopathy* (CMO) is a periosteal proliferation along the body of the mandible, and it can be extensive enough to incorporate the temporomandibular joint. Some discomfort may be present, which can be managed with anti-inflammatory agents, but no specific therapy is recommended. Regression usually occurs by 11 to 13 months of age, with a few patients having only partial recovery.

Injury

Any time an injury to the teeth is noticed, the facial bones should also be evaluated and vice versa. Trauma to the facial bones can cause fractures (simple to complicated), temporomandibular joint *luxation,* or even the avulsion of structures. Specific information on the type and location of a fracture as related to appropriate treatment will be covered in chapter 6: Oral and Dental Emergencies.

Neoplasia

Primary osseous neoplasia (osteosarcoma) is not common in the mandible and maxilla, but other tumors extending from oral soft tissues often greatly affect the underlying bone. In fact, locally aggressive characteristics, including osseous involvement and frequent recurrence, are the hallmark of many oral tumors, including SCC, *fibrosarcoma,* and even acanthomatous epulides (see the section on oral and dental tumors at the end of this chapter).

Systemic Diseases

Other diseases that affect bones in the body can also affect the bones of the oral cavity. Hyperparathyroidism, whether primary or secondary to renal failure or inappropriate diet, causes a demineralization of the bone, resulting in a *"rubber jaw,"* wherein the osseous tissue becomes very soft. Infectious diseases involving fungi or bacteria can also result in osteomyelitis, though many forms of infection occur because of a local infectious agent present in or introduced into the oral cavity.

TMJ Locking

If head trauma has occurred to an animal, open mouth locking is often attributable to the luxation of the TMJ. In the absence of head trauma, if there is luxation of the TMJ, some form of TMJ dysplasia is probably present, with sufficient laxity to allow a subluxation of the joint (particularly when the mouth is wide open) so the coronoid process of the mandible of the opposite side can "slip out" laterally under the ridge of the zygomatic arch and become stuck there. Therapy of the affected joint is usually not successful, but reduction of the zygomatic arch or coronoid process helps prevent the locking from recurring.

Lips

Lips are the most obvious aspect of the oral cavity, but lip lesions can sometimes be covered by hair and are occasionally overlooked. Abnormalities of the lips can, at times, be attributed to oral problems, or they may be an extension of external skin problems. As a significant mucocutaneous junction, this area is sometimes the site of specific immune problems.

Chelitis

Chelitis is a general term for an inflammation of the lips, resulting from a wide variety of causes. Autoimmune diseases involving the mucocutaneous junction should be biopsied for proper diagnosis. Inflammatory oral disease may extend to the lips and deposit excessive amounts of saliva in the region, resulting in a pyoderma. Lip-fold pyoderma in some breeds with pendulous lips can be difficult to control.

Eosinophilic Granuloma Complex

"Rodent ulcer" (or *indolent ulcer*), found in some cats, is one form of eosinophilic granuloma that can develop on the upper lip. Any suspicious lesion should be biopsied to rule out neoplasia or an autoimmune disorder.

Cleft Lip or Palate

A congenital lesion of cleft lip with extension to the palate to one side of the rostral midline is considered a primary palatal cleft. Acquired lesions may result from injury, including those caused by chewing on electrical cords.

Tight Lip

   A Chinese shar pei may have a condition in which there is minimal space between the mandibular teeth and the lip (vestibular space). The condition can become severe enough to force the lower lip over the incisors and canines (Figure 2.14). Chronic irritation and infection may occur if the lip interferes with proper mouth closing. Repair involves deepening the vestibular space in the region to loosen the lip.

Palate

   The roof of the mouth provides a distinct division between the oral cavity and the nose rostral to the pharynx. Any disruption in the palate can lead to chronic fistulation between the cavities.

Congenital Defects

   As discussed in the section on the lip, a primary *cleft palate* involves the rostral region, lateral to the midline (Figure 2.15). This corresponds to the y-shaped suture line of fusion of the incisive bone to the paired maxillae. A midline palate defect caudal to this area is a secondary palate. Such a defect can cause problems in nursing for infants, and repair is often necessary.

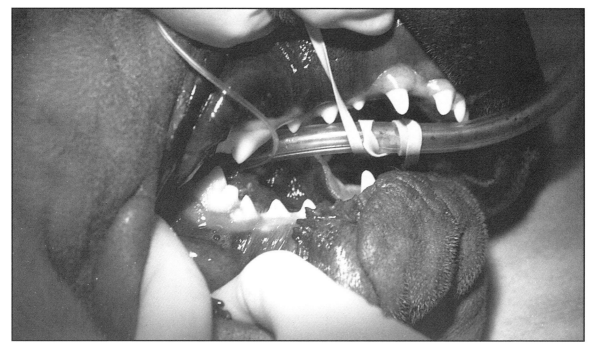

Figure 2.14 *Tight lip in a Chinese shar pei*

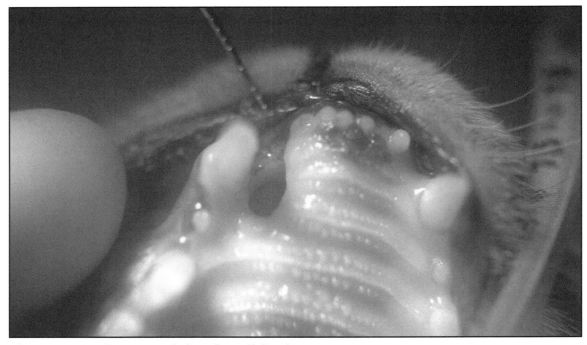

Figure 2.15 *Primary cleft palate (feline)*

Acquired Defects

Acquired defects may result from trauma (e.g., falling from a high-rise building, being hit by a car and splitting the palate, or chewing on an electrical cord) or even extensive periodontal disease (oronasal or oroantral fistulation). Traumatic injury from sharp objects or foreign bodies may also damage the palate without causing an extreme loss of tissue.

Inflammation

The palate can show an extension of periodontal disease, particularly in severe cases of lymphocytic-plasmacytic stomatitis in cats. Such an inflammation may be apparent only as a "red-line" lesion, or it may be as involved as a proliferative growth of tissue. Autoimmune diseases may also be evident as a palatal lesion, as can tumors, which require biopsy for an accurate diagnosis.

Salivary Glands and Ducts

Additional knowledge of the location of salivary ducts and glands, as well as specific methods for evaluation (sialography), may be necessary to fully evaluate abnormalities.

Ranula or Mucocele

If the proper flow of saliva is disrupted, the pooling of secretions can cause a very large swelling (Figure 2.16). At times, tying off of the duct can lead to disuse atrophy, but either removal or marsupialization is often necessary to allow the saliva to drain directly into the oral cavity.

Neoplasia

Neoplasia of the salivary gland is not common, but it can be encountered in domestic pets. Adequate biopsy to differentiate it from inflammation (sialodenitis) may be necessary.

Neuromuscular Structures

Though most of the oral musculature is actually located outside the oral cavity proper, without it, the cavity could not function properly.

Atrophy

Disuse atrophy of the oral musculature is always a possibility in animals, but virtually the only situation in which it occurs is when an animal is being fed by alternate means. Typically, atrophy of the muscles of mastication is due to innervation problems.

Masticatory Muscle Myositis

A rather specific syndrome with immune ramifications, masticatory muscle myositis (MMM) manifests itself in a pet who has great difficulty in opening its mouth, without osseous causes. Blood work to detect type-2M muscle autoantibodies can be used to confirm a diagnosis, though biopsy is sometimes needed to fully evaluate the pet's status.

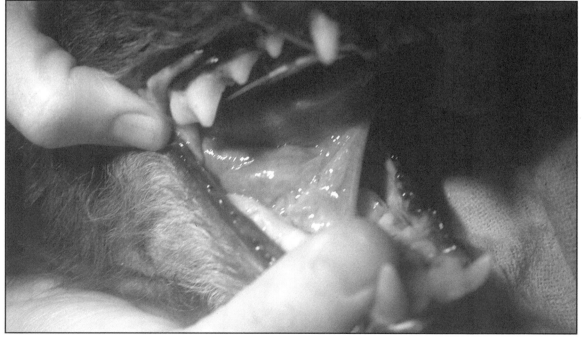

Figure 2.16 *Sublingual ranula*

Mandibular Neuropraxia

In a dog with a history of carrying large objects in its mouth, a dropped-open mouth may signify stress affecting the nerves that supply the masticatory muscles. Rest and supportive therapy usually result in recovery.

ORAL AND DENTAL TUMORS

Because many oral tumors in dogs and cats can be extremely aggressive, with local infiltration or metastasis, regular oral examination is essential for early detection. With some early lesions, immediate and appropriate therapy may at least give the patient a chance for survival, depending on tumor type, location, and staging.

Dogs

The three most common malignant tumors in the dog are malignant melanomas, fibrosarcomas, and squamous cell carcinomas. Other malignant tumors such as osteosarcomas, mastocytomas, and lymphosarcomas are, at times, found in the oral cavity. Benign tumors such as papillomas seldom cause problems, but odontogenic tumors and cysts can sometimes affect adjacent tissue.

Malignant Melanomas

Found in the gingiva, mucosa, palate, and tongue, melanomas tend to be the most aggressive tumors in the oral cavity, often having metastasized by the time of detection. Predilection is in older, darker-pigmented dogs, more frequently in males. These tumors vary in appearance, including the degree of pigmentation (Plate 4). Aggressive surgery with ancillary therapy may be helpful if the melanoma is caught early.

Squamous Cell Carcinomas

Squamous cell carcinomas can be found almost anywhere in the oral cavity, with the tonsillar form carrying the worst prognosis. Nontonsillar SCC can be locally invasive but is slow to metastasize, and there is a better prognosis for those lesions located further rostrally in the mouth. Extension into bone tissue is common. Wide excision, with or without radiation, therapy can sometimes be effective (Plates 5 and 6).

Fibrosarcomas

The third most common tumors in the dog, fibrosarcomas are more often seen in the larger breeds. They sometimes have a rapid local invasion into bone, as well as a high recurrence rate, though they metastasize slowly. The maxillary gingiva and palate are frequent sites for these tumors, which may initially appear benign. Early detection and aggressive resection at that point improve the prognosis.

Cats

Squamous cell carcinoma is by far the most common oral neoplasia in cats, followed by fibrosarcoma and melanosarcoma. Benign growths are uncommon in cats, but an occasional *epulis* or nasopharyngeal polyp can be found.

Squamous Cell Carcinomas

As in the dog, these tumors are locally invasive and slow to metastasize in cats, except for the more aggressive tonsillar form. The tongue (including the sublingual area) and gingiva are frequent sites. SCC of the mandible can be treated favorably with hemimandibulectomy.

Fibrosarcomas

Occasionally seen in the cat, the biological behavior of these tumors are as described earlier—slow to metastasize, locally invasive, and frequently recurring. For adequate resection, early detection is very important.

Malignant Melanomas

Rarely seen in the cat, malignant melanomas most often have metastasized by the time of detection. Aggressive surgery with adjunct therapy may prolong life expectation.

CHAPTER 3

Periodontal Disease

According to the *Guinness World Book of Records,* periodontal disease is the most common infectious disease of man. This seems to hold true for our domestic pets as well. Studies have shown the tremendous prevalence of periodontal disease in the general pet population, emphasizing the need to adequately treat such a widespread problem.

PATHOGENESIS

Understanding the progression of periodontal disease, with its cyclical nature of active inflammation and quiescence, will help you determine the best course of action. Each patient—in fact, each individual tooth—needs separate evaluation, as you may encounter many variations of periodontal disease.

Bacteria

Though many factors play a role in this problem, without bacteria there would be no periodontal disease, which makes it an infectious problem. The microorganisms mix with salivary glycoproteins and extracellular polysaccharides to form the soft, sticky plaque that adheres to the tooth surface. If left there, the plaque eventually converts into calculus when it becomes mineralized. The soft plaque is the most "active" phase, with the bacteria starting out as gram-positive, nonmotile aerobic cocci on the supragingival surfaces. Contact with the gingiva stimulates an inflammatory response in the body to fight the bacteria. Continued deposition of plaque, along with the formation of calculus, leads to significant deposits. As this continues, the deeper layers of this biofilm convert to anaerobic, gram-negative, motile rods and filamentous organisms that are more virulent with endotoxins. Continued bacterial presence leads to the direct toxic effects of inflammation and even loss of tissue.

Host Defenses

The body's first line of defense when dealing with bacteria in the oral cavity is usually to move neutrophils into the affected areas. Immune responses are also common in the oral cavity. In most healthy animals, there is a reasonable balance in the host response to bacterial insult.

In some individuals, however, the protective response of the body may be excessive. Although the bacteria may have a restricted "range," in terms of how far a direct effect on tissues might take them, a humoral and cellular response from the patient can end up destroying more tissue than the bacteria ever would have.

Attachment Loss

From both the direct influence of bacteria on the tissues and the host's defense mechanism, the most significant aspect of periodontal disease is the loss of periodontal attachment that occurs without proper therapy. With compromised support, teeth can be lost.

Attached Gingiva

As stated earlier, attached gingiva is the rim of gingiva located closest to the crown, with distinct connective tissue ties to the underlying bone. This gingiva is the periodontal tissue's first line of defense, so it is imperative to try to preserve at least 2 to 3 mm of attached gingiva while minimizing pocket depth (Plate 7).

Alveolar Bone

Providing support to the remaining periodontal structures, the alveolar bone provides a solid structure to house the roots of teeth. Bone loss typically is first evident radiographically with a loss of distinction of the alveolar crest, the ridge of bone between teeth (and roots). Because the direct effect of bacteria and bacterial by-products can only radiate a limited distance, it is the progression of attachment loss (and progressive movement) and the introduction of bacteria into the deeper tissues that allows additional loss of structures, if left unchecked. Host defenses against the bacteria can cause even greater damage and attachment loss, to the point of excess in some cases.

Horizontal Bone Loss. Once crestal bone is lost, additional destruction of bone can occur in one of two basic ways or through a combination of the two. In generalized *periodontitis,* with involvement of multiple teeth, the overall level or height of bone is lost in a horizontal manner. The pockets generally do not extend into a defect between the tooth and bone (see the section vertical bone loss below), so they are considered to be *suprabony pockets.*

Vertical Bone Loss. Focal bone loss can occur down the length of a root, sometimes causing a deep, well-like defect. This vertical bone loss often results in a pocket between the tooth and the alveolar bone, known as an *intrabony* or *infrabony pocket* (Figure 3.1). There may be from one to four bony "walls" of the defect, depending on the pattern of bone loss around the root.

Consequences of Attachment Loss

The eventual consequences of soft- and hard-tissue loss result in a variety of clinical problems. If the general height of the gingiva remains the same but there is a loss of *epithelial attachment,* periodontal ligament, and bone, there will be deep pockets that are identified initially through periodontal probing and further evaluated radiographically. Such deep pockets often exhibit more vertical bone loss, though they can be present in multiple foci. These pockets allow a progressive destruction of deeper layers if adequate therapy is not performed.

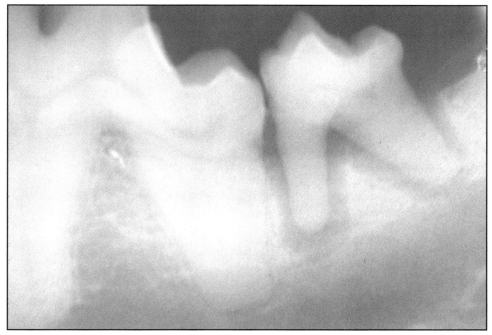

Figure 3.1 *Complete vertical bone loss in a mandibular second molar*

A more linear form of tissue loss results as the level of gingiva and bone retreats, causing gingival recession and horizontal bone loss with root exposure and eventual exposure of the furcation of multirooted teeth. There may be minimal pocket depths, but the loss of attached gingiva should be minimized (2 to 3 mm at a minimum) for protection. An exposure of furcation areas, although manageable with adequate home care, can cause complications because of the retention of food and plaque; it may also make it difficult to adequately clean all affected surfaces, particularly in the three-rooted upper fourth premolars and molars. In addition, the development of deep pockets in such a situation can result in significant total attachment loss, mobility, and even tooth loss.

STAGES OF PERIODONTAL DISEASE

It is helpful to be able to categorize the level of periodontal disease for record keeping, client and veterinarian communication, and treatment planning and assessment. The extent or stage of periodontal disease is based primarily on the loss of attachment as the tissues of the periodontium (gingiva, periodontal ligament [PDL], cementum, alveolar bone) are destroyed. You can use many other indexes in dentistry to indicate levels of plaque and calculus accumulation, degree of gingival inflammation, mobility, and so on to further describe the pathology present.

Table 3.1
Stages of periodontal disease

Stage	Description	Attachment loss (%)
0	Normal	0
1	Gingivitis	0
2	Early periodontitis	< 25
3	Moderate periodontitis	> 25
4	Severe periodontitis	> 50

Because periodontal disease itself is a cyclic disease, with periods of activity and dormancy, examination at any one time may tell just part of the story. Active inflammation may not be marked in an area where there is extensive attachment loss. However, because the loss is present, the potential for future inflammation is always there. In evaluating a therapeutic response, the regular absence of inflammation posttreatment, even with significant areas of attachment loss, may indicate some level of control over the active phases of the disease.

In addition, different areas of the mouth may exhibit varying stages of periodontal disease (see Table 3.1.) You should treat patients with this type of periodontal disease on a site-by-site basis, making an overall evaluation for generalized patterns. The next section will cover basic characteristics of the stages of periodontal disease, including bacterial involvement, extent of attachment loss, and basic therapy theory. Details on appropriate treatments will be covered in the section on periodontal therapy.

Stage I Periodontal Disease: Gingivitis

Stage I periodontal disease, gingivitis, exhibits the following characteristics:

Bacteria
The bacteria in stage I periodontal disease stays primarily in the supragingival area, so they are generally aerobic. Gram-positive cocci (nonmotile) are the most common forms found; these bacteria have lower levels of virulence.

Attachment
This earliest stage of periodontal disease involves the initial inflammation of the *gingival margin,* with no deeper inflammation or attachment loss. There may be an increase in sulcus depth, but this is primarily caused by an increase in the free gingival margin, as it can be edematous with inflammation. With no attachment loss, this is the only stage of periodontal disease that is reversible.

Therapy
The primary treatment goals for periodontal disease are to remove all biofilm (plaque, calculus, debris) and to minimize attachment loss. *Prophylaxis,* which means "prevention," is really a preventative only at this stage of the disease, when the inflammation is still reversible and no attachment has yet been lost.

Stage II Periodontal Disease: Early Periodontitis

Stage II periodontal disease, early periodontitis, exhibits the following characteristics:

Bacteria

With the accumulation of additional supragingival plaque and calculus, the opening to the sulcus becomes occluded, restricting oxygen flow to the sulcus region. Adding this to increased pocket depth caused by attachment loss, the bacteria in the subgingival recessions start to change to more anaerobic strains—gram-negative rods with increasing levels of virulence.

Attachment Loss

Stage II periodontal disease encompasses those teeth with up to 25% attachment loss. The first evidence of the loss of periodontal support may be increasing pocket depth. This may initially stem from the loss of integrity of the attachment of the junctional epithelium to the tooth at the base of the pocket, allowing the probe to slip through to deeper levels. This progresses to actual soft-tissue loss of the epithelium and underlying periodontal ligament. With enough bacterial involvement and host response, crestal bone starts to deteriorate, which is often the first detectable radiographic sign.

Therapy

In addition to completing the basic steps of a dental cleaning, pay close attention to the developing pocket. At this stage, you can use *curettes* or appropriate subgingival ultrasonic instruments effectively to clean the root surfaces without having to raise a gingival flap, with a technique called closed *root planing* (in pockets up to 5 mm). Calculus and debris left in the pocket will only predispose the area to further involvement. Medications (perioceutics) can be placed in the pockets to enhance therapy. Regular dental cleanings and home care are even more vital at this stage to prevent a progression of the attachment loss that could endanger the teeth.

Stage III Periodontal Disease: Moderate Periodontitis

Stage III periodontal disease exhibits the following characteristics:

Bacteria

With the development of deeper pockets, the abundance of anaerobic microbes flourishes. Routine home care or oral rinses cannot reach these areas, so the bacteria can extend into underlying tissue, even causing alveolitis or osteomyelitis. The gram-negative colonies can be more virulent mobile rods, spirochetes, and fusiform bacteria. Though specific antibiotic therapy, even in a pulse regimen, can help bring down the numbers of bacteria present, the disease will continue to progress unless the bacteria and biofilm are removed.

Attachment Loss

In stage III lesions, up to 50% of the attachment may be lost. This is a significant percentage of the integral support of the tooth, and such a loss can greatly threaten the tooth's retention. Close attention to the evaluation of pocket depth, the amount of attached gingiva, the level of bone height, and the characteristics of the defect (infrabony or suprabony, number of bony walls in pocket, furcation involvement, etc.) will help you plan treatment.

Therapy

Once you have evaluated the preceding factors, therapy can be instituted. For example, if the loss involves both soft and hard tissue, there can be significant root and furcation exposure, with minimal pocket depth. In such cases, a thorough cleaning of the exposed surfaces is vital, but there may be only a minimal need for pocket therapy. If primarily bone is lost, particularly in a horizontal manner and with no evidence of infrabony pockets, the primary therapy will be to clean the tooth surfaces and treat the soft-tissue pockets. Treatment of specific infrabony pockets involves cleaning the areas and potentially considering regenerative therapy to influence the regrowth of bone to increase support and attachment. Owner commitment to regular professional care and good home care is essential.

Stage IV Periodontal Disease: Severe Periodontitis

Stage IV periodontal disease exhibits the following characteristics:

Bacteria

The general bacterial population in this stage will be similar to that described in the section on stage III periodontal disease.

Attachment Loss

Teeth in this category, with more than 50% attachment loss, must be thoroughly evaluated because the salvagability of the tooth may be in question. Initially, an accurate assessment of bone level, pocket depth, attached gingiva, and mobility should be made.

Therapy

The first step in treatment planning is deciding whether to save the tooth, which must be done almost on an individual basis. Many factors play a part in this decision, including your skill level and the commitment of the owner to providing adequate home care and regular professional therapy. The relative importance of the tooth ("strategic" versus "nonstrategic" teeth) plays a part as well, as retention of a canine or *carnassial* tooth may be more significant than retention of an incisor or smaller premolar. The general health of the animal is also very important to assess, as longer, multiple anesthetic episodes may be necessary for regenerative procedures. Some patients might be better off having the teeth extracted in order to remove a potential source of bacteria that could enter the bloodstream.

This may be particularly vital in high-risk patients with valvular disease, organ disease or immunosuppression, or in those with prosthetic implants.

In some highly strategic teeth, where tooth loss could compromise bone stability (lower first molar or canine, upper canine with bone loss encroaching upon the nasal cavity), saving the tooth and improving the bone integrity is the optimum goal. Any regenerative attempt should not be considered lightly, for it will take a strong combination of skill on your part, reasonable risk levels for multiple anesthetic episodes, and a dedicated owner.

PERIODONTAL COMPLICATIONS

Because there is a wide range of manifestations of periodontal disease and a host of potential individual responses, you may, on occasion, find some severe forms of the disease or sequela of attachment loss. In these cases, routine therapy may be insufficient to handle the problems encountered.

Refractory Periodontitis

Refractory periodontitis is one form of severe periodontal disease and has a variety of presentations.

Stomatitis (Lymphocytic-Plasmacytic)

Covered more thoroughly in chapter 7: Feline Oral and Dental Disease, this range of syndromes basically indicates an excessive host defense response that is inappropriate to the level of plaque and calculus accumulation. Viral and bacterial components may be contributing factors, but the exact etiology is unknown.

Chronic Ulcerative Paradental Stomatitis (CUPS)

Sometimes described as "kissing ulcers," these lesions are generally located on mucosal surfaces that contact tooth surfaces covered with accumulations of plaque and calculus (Plate 8). Again, it is typically the individual's excessive host response that leads to these lesions ("plaque intolerance"). Meticulous oral care may lessen their severity, but sometimes extraction is the only answer. Some individuals may experience improvement with a concurrent use of sulcal perioceutics (HESKA PERIOceutic GEL) at the time of periodontal therapy.

Juvenile Periodontitis

Although the refractory periodontitis conditions described thus far occur most frequently in adult animals, occasionally a younger animal will exhibit inappropriate levels of inflammatory gingival tissue. In some of these cases, regular cleaning and home care to minimize the degree of attachment loss can get the animal through this stage until further maturity. Certain individuals actually "grow out" of the inflammatory stage, and if there has been minimal attachment loss, they can then maintain relatively healthy teeth. By contrast, some breeds, particularly in cats (Abysinnians, etc.), maintain an inflammatory state even after reaching maturity.

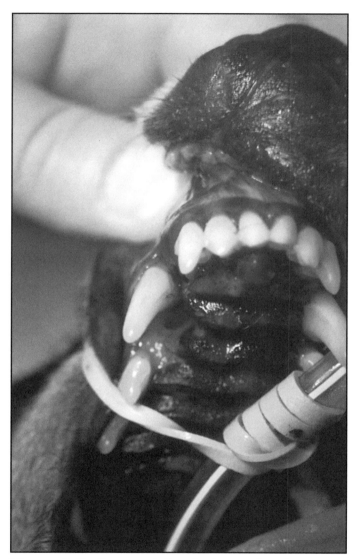

Figure 3.2 *Oronasal fistulation, palatal aspect of a maxillary canine*

Autoimmune Diseases

Pemphigoid-type diseases often have visible signs in the oral cavity—indeed, sometimes these are the first signs (Plate 9). In cases of nonresponsive, ulcerative stomatitis (especially palatitis and cheilitis), take a biopsy to rule out an autoimmune cause. If an autoimmune condition is diagnosed, regular dental care with immunosuppressive therapy is often needed. Other body systems should be thoroughly evaluated for additional involvement.

Oronasal and Oroantral Fistulation

With the maxillary teeth, the width of alveolar bone between the teeth and the nasal cavity or sinus (antral) can often be fairly thin, particularly in long, narrow-nosed dogs such as dachshunds. Given that and the relative obscurity of oronasal and oroantral fistulations (which are palatally located), it is not surprising that significant amounts of bone loss often go undetected until eventual fistulation into the nasal passages (Figure 3.2). Even then, without proper probing and evaluation, such lesions often go undiagnosed until there is tooth loss and fistula exposure, even when a chronic nasal discharge or sinusitis is present.

On top of that, with the unique problem caused by the constant strain of respiratory pressures against the suture line of a repair, specific methods of oronasal fistulation—oroantral fistulation (ONF-OAF) closure must be used (see chapter 4: Oral Surgery). Yet even with good surgical technique, the potential for dehiscence or persistence of an opening exists. Additional surgery may be necessary, but ideally it would be needed only to close much smaller defects.

Pathologic Fractures

When there is a significant amount of periodontal bone loss, particularly in the mandible, there can be enough compromise of the bone to predispose it to a pathological fracture with minor traumatic forces. This is most frequently seen at the sites of the lower first molars (mandibular body fractures) and the canines (symphyseal fractures).

Because the bone is already endangered by the bone loss and extractions are probably needed, adequate fixation and healing of these sites are often difficult. Preventing this condition is definitely the preferred course. Periodontal bone loss around incisors may also predispose these teeth to avulsion by chewing, playing tug-of-war, and so forth.

Periodontal Abscesses

When bacteria or infected debris remains trapped in a deep periodontal pocket, possibly due to inadequate flushing after therapy, a periodontal abscess may result. The draining tract of the fistula will generally open below the mucogingival line, in the region of the attached gingiva (Plate 10). Without proper treatment, the fistula will cause progressive attachment loss. If not draining, the abscess may need to be lanced, either through the gingiva or up into the sulcus.

Periodontal-Endodontic Disease

When the bone loss occurs in a vertical fashion and is unchecked, to the point at which the apical region is involved, bacteria can get into the root canal system and infect the pulpal tissues. After the pulp dies, a periapical abscess can then develop at the other apex (or apexes) of multirooted teeth. Such a condition is difficult to treat because both endodontic (root canal) therapy and periodontal surgery would be needed to salvage the entire tooth, so extraction is often recommended. Resecting the periodontal-affected root and performing endodontic therapy of the other root(s) can save a part of the tooth that might still have a healthy peridontium (Figure 3.3). Primary endodontic disease with periapical infection can progress up a root to compromise the attachment in endodontic-periodontic disease.

PERIODONTAL THERAPY

There are four main goals in providing adequate periodontal therapy for optimal periodontal health: removing biofilm (plaque, calculus, debris); minimizing attachment loss; minimizing pocket depth; and maintaining a minimum of attached gingiva (2 to 3 mm). The most common term used for treatment, *prophylaxis,* is typically a misnomer. Seldom is a "dental cleaning" simply that—prevention. Usually, there is additional salvage work to do. The term *periodontal therapy* is much more accurate and more professional.

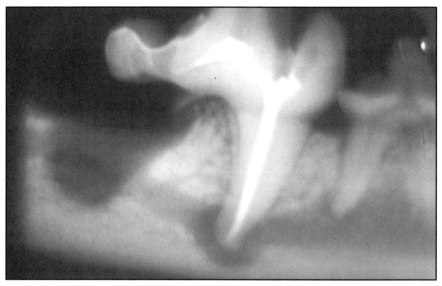

Figure 3.3 *Periodontic-endodontic lesion: Periodontal bone loss of distal root (mandibular first molar) extended into pulp system, causing periapical bone loss at mesial root; distal root was resected, and mesial root was treated with endodontic therapy*

Antibiotics

The use of antibiotics can play an important role in the treatment of periodontal disease because it is an infection process caused by bacteria. Each case should be evaluated individually as to the indication for and choice of antibiotic. For most routine prophylaxes with minimal to moderate calculus and minimal attachment loss in a healthy patient, the transient bacteremia generally does not pose a significant problem. Exception would be those individuals with predisposing conditions that warrant antibacterial protection to reduce the potential risks of bacteremia (e.g., patients with heart conditions, prosthetic devices, organ diseases). Antibiotic coverage from 1 hour prior to the procedure extending up to 6 hours afterward is usually sufficient. In heavily infected mouths, oral antibiotics started a few days prior to therapy can result in significant clinical improvement and a more accurate picture of the periodontal status once the inflammation has subsided. Some patients might experience such an improvement that the client may be tempted to delay therapy, so always encourage follow-through on therapeutic recommendations. Although a pulse therapy of antibiotics may make the pet feel better by moderating the bacterial load, it should never be a substitute for complete treatment. In addition, if an animal has been on one particular antibiotic for whatever reason for a period of time, it may be advisable to change or add to the antibiotic to cover any possible resistant strains. Postoperative antibiotics may be extended to help resolve infections such as abscesses or alveolitis once the initial therapy is complete.

Complete "Prophylaxis"

Some clients may be hesitant about anesthetizing their pets. However, it is essential to use full general anesthesia (with a cuffed endotracheal tube in place), and have operator protection as well (mask, eye protection, gloves), given the aerosolization of bacteria during the procedure. Preanesthetic workups and appropriate anesthesia protocol and monitoring can minimize the risks in order to realize the benefits the therapy can afford.

Steps

Some of your clients may object to the cost of dental therapy. However, if you discuss anesthesia costs with them and give them with a detailed description of the steps of a complete "prophy" (verbally, via a handout, or both), you can effectively inform them about the individualized attention their pet will receive.

This individualized care will incorporate the following steps:

- Supragingival scaling
- Subgingival scaling
- Charting
- Polishing
- Irrigation
- Fluoride application
- Additional procedures:
    — Root planing
    — Subgingival curettage
    — Ultrasonic periodontal debridement
    — Radiography
    — Advanced periodontal therapy, including perioceutics, gingival flaps, regenerative therapy, and splinting

Supragingival Scaling. Gross removal of plaque and calculus from the crown surfaces (supragingival) is the first step. Unfortunately, because this first step greatly improves the appearance of the teeth, some owners may consider this adequate therapy—but it is far from that!

You can use most forms of scalers on these surfaces (hoes, hand scalers, ultrasonic scalers, etc.). The use of calculus forceps to remove large pieces of calculus can greatly speed up the procedure. Just be careful not to accidentally fracture a crown or to "extract" any teeth that are being held in by a bridge of calculus!

Ultrasonic Scalers. Probably the most common scaler used in veterinary practices, this piece of equipment must be used correctly to avoid damaging the teeth. The tip can overheat due to the frequency of the vibrating stacks, so adequate water flow to the tip is essential. In some scalers, the side (not the tip) should be used on any one tooth for no more than 12 to 15 seconds at a time, with a light touch. If the tip gets too hot to hold in your fingertips, you should change it or put it aside until cool—do other work, such as hand scaling, charting, and so forth. Excessive heat applied to the tooth can cause pulpal hyperthermia, inflammation, and even death of the pulp. A pinkish tint that eventually fades may indicate a reversible form of pulpitis, but a dark-purple or gray tooth is likely nonvital (see chapter 5: Advanced Oral and Dental Problems—Endodontics).

Rotary Scalers. A six-sided, soft-steel bur can be used on an air-driven, *high-speed handpiece* for rapid removal of calculus by "vibrating" it off. If used incorrectly, however, rotary scaling can cause significant tooth damage both directly to the enamel and by hyperthermic damage to the pulp. Burs must be sharp to be effective, and because they dull quickly, you should replace them on a regular basis. A dull bur will not effectively remove calculus, so the inexperienced operator will often use more force to achieve desired results, possibly damaging the tooth in the process.

Sonic Scalers. These scalers are used on a high-speed handpiece port to generate a lower-frequency vibration (as compared to sonic scalers) that produces minimal heat. Sufficient air-compressor capacity is needed to get 35 to 40 psi to the scaler for optimum efficiency. Water spray is used primarily for irrigation and not as a coolant. The main drawback with this equipment is the cost of the scaler and the lack of power if sufficient pressure is not available.

Subgingival Scaling. No matter how clean a crown is, the full process of periodontal disease can continue in the sulcus if you leave debris there. You should avoid the use of most rotary- and standard-tip ultrasonic scalers because of the damage they can do (hyperthermia, lack of irrigant at the tip). Some ultrasonics scalers are specifically designed for subgingival scaling, and sonic scalers can be used carefully; hand scaling can provide gentler cleaning as well as tactile feedback.

Hand Instruments (Curettes). To properly treat subgingival regions, hand instruments called curettes are the equipment of choice. With a rounded toe and back (half-moon shape in cross section), this device can be introduced into the depth of the sulcus with minimal damage to the tissues. Use a Modified Pen Grasp to grip the instrument, with the middle finger on the lower handle and the index finger and thumb providing a balanced force. The ring finger serves as a fulcrum for a wrist-rocking motion. A scaler, with pointed tip and back (triangular in cross section), should only be used supragingivally. Most curettes have one "cutting edge" on each working head, often a mirror image of the opposite end, so the same instrument can be used on different surfaces of the tooth.

Once placed to the depth of the pocket, the cutting edge is turned to engage the surface of the tooth. The instrument is drawn out of the pocket along the surface of the tooth in a pull stroke to dislodge calculus deposits and debris. A series of overlapping strokes (vertical, oblique, etc.) can clean all areas in a crosshatch pattern. A hand curette can effectively reach as far as 5 mm (with adequate visualization) without raising a gingival flap. You must keep curettes sharpened for maximum effectiveness (see chapter 9: Materials and Equipment).

Charting. Throughout the process of cleaning, you should continuously evaluate the periodontal status. Set aside a specific time for recording any irregularities encountered, including gingival recession, root or furcation exposure, pocket formation, tooth fracture, resorptive lesions, mobility, and the like. Ideally, probe each tooth at six locations (buccal and lingual or palatal, then four *line angles* at the "corners"—mesial-buccal, etc.). A more practical method is to gently insert the probe into the sulcus and "walk" it around the tooth, charting any significant pocket depths, root exposure, and so forth. There are many types of charts, stickers, and other means of record keeping: Just be consistent with your method, and be sure it can be accurately interpreted. Specific dental records not only provide good medical documentation, they also provide an excellent means for evaluating tissue response to therapy on subsequent exams.

Polishing. Any time a tooth surface is scaled, even if hand scaled, microscopic scratches occur on the enamel. Plaque can attach to a smooth tooth surface 30 minutes after a complete cleaning, and a rougher surface will allow an even more rapid accumulation, which can be more difficult to remove at future cleanings. Polishing with a fine to medium pumice can help smooth the surfaces when done correctly. Some pumices also contain fluoride, but use only flour pumice if additional dentin bonding or restorative procedures are to be done.

Improper polishing, with inadequate amounts of prophy paste, excessive pressure, or prolonged time spent on teeth, can cause damage to the tooth from hyperthermia. Prophy angle speeds should not exceed 3,000 rpm; with variable speed units, speed should be kept at a minimum to avoid potential damage.

Irrigation. Once the teeth are completely cleaned and polished, gently and thoroughly flush the tooth surfaces and pockets to remove all loose debris, including prophy paste. Any material left behind can result in continued periodontal inflammation or even an abscess. The most convenient method is to use the three-way air and water syringe on an air-driven unit, with a moderate water stream. Use the air stream to blow the surfaces dry, which helps to expose any residual debris (a calculus appears chalky). Other methods of irrigation include the use of urinary catheters or blunt-nosed needles on large syringes. With these methods, you can apply medicaments, such as dilute chlorhexidine or fluoride, for a final antimicrobial rinse.

Fluoride. Although there has been some debate over the use of fluoride and although toxicity can be a problem if it is used unwisely or if inappropriate amounts are ingested, fluoride can be a useful adjunct to periodontal therapy when properly employed. Fluoride is antibacterial and can also help with sensitive teeth, particularly if exposed roots have been cleaned.

Many types and forms of fluoride are available, with different indications. In general, those used "postprophy" are applied to a dry tooth surface and wiped or blown off (never rinsed!), so moisture is not a factor. Sodium fluorides are effectively used in this manner, in viscous gels or foams that are applied directly to the tooth surface. Use home-care fluorides with the assumption that moisture will be present, so stannous fluoride will often be your choice.

Additional Procedures: Root Planing. The use of curettes has already been briefly described (see the section on subgingival scaling) as a method to clean tooth surfaces in a pocket or deep sulcus. With more extensive attachment loss, particularly with root exposure, pay specific attention these areas. The term *root planing* is commonly used to describe the scaling method of cross-hatching strokes, as well as periodontal debridement (a term also used with certain periodontal scaling systems). If the pocket is 5 mm or less and the curette is of sufficient size to reach the pocket depth, closed-root planing can typically be effective. Any pockets deeper than that require better access to the area, achieved by raising a gingival flap to expose the area for scaling, a procedure that is known as open-root planing. This exposure is of particular importance when treating deep vertical pockets or doing regenerative therapy because all debris and even granulation tissue must be thoroughly debrided in such cases. (Specific therapy will be covered in the next section.)

Subgingival Curettage. In closed-root planing procedures, also use the curette to gently debride the inner surface of the gingiva to remove bacteria and necrotic debris. By slightly changing the angle of the working head (to engage the soft tissue) and placing light digital pressure on the outside, draw the curette up along the soft tissue to "scrape" it clean.

Radiography

Of course, for a full evaluation and to assess any degree of attachment loss, oral radiographs can be indispensable. With radiographs, you can correlate the level of attachment loss with the bone height to classify the pocket type (suprabony or infrabony) and determine the extent of damage (stage of disease). Additional problems may become evident on radiographs (periodontal-endodontic lesion, abnormal bone, etc.).

Advanced Periodontal Therapy

The common goals of periodontal therapy are to remove the biofilm while preserving attached gingiva and minimizing pocket depth and attachment loss. The actual therapy will vary depending on pocket depth, type of pocket (suprabony or infrabony), and desired outcome (salvage versus extraction).

Pockets up to 5 mm

Shallow pockets may be treated with one of several approaches including closed-root planing, perioceutics, and improved home care.

Closed-Root Planing. You can often treat more shallow pockets without having to raise a gingival flap (Figure 3.4). Closed-root planing with subgingival curettage (see previous section) will typically suffice to clean the region. Most pockets of this depth will be primarily soft tissue in nature (suprabony), though some extension into alveolar bone is possible.

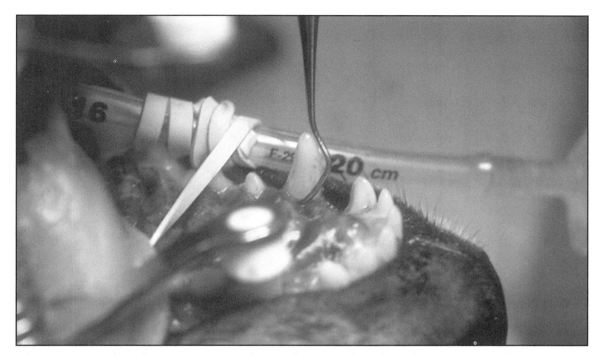

Figure 3.4 *Closed-root planing of a moderate palatal pocket in a maxillary canine*

Perioceutics. In addition to techniques for removing all biofilm and necrotic debris, new therapies known as perioceutics are now available to implant medicaments into the periodontal pockets. One such product, the HESKA PERIOceutic GEL (Heska, Fort Collins, CO), consists of doxycycline mixed into a biodegradable gel that is "injected" into the sulcus or pocket (Figure 3.5). Once solidified (water speeds up the process), the gel is packed into the pocket with the plastic packing instrument provided or a metal W-3 instrument (which sticks less to the gel than the plastic instrument does). Once in place, the gel releases doxycycline directly into the pocket, at higher levels than systemic doses of the antibiotic could release into the gingival crevicular fluid (GCF). In this way, an effective dose of the antibiotic can be administered where it is needed locally, without having to give it systemically. Doxycycline, like other tetracycline products, also has an anticollagenolytic effect, which can moderate the destructive processes of periodontal disease.

Home Care. Every periodontal therapy can be enhanced with proper home care to reduce bacterial load and plaque formation. Stage more advanced procedures with the initial therapy of cleaning and perioceutics, followed by home care; this will not only allow the tissues to become healthier and less inflamed but will also let you assess the level of commitment the owner may or may not have. Lack of adherence to home care and recheck schedules may worsen the prognosis of effective treatment.

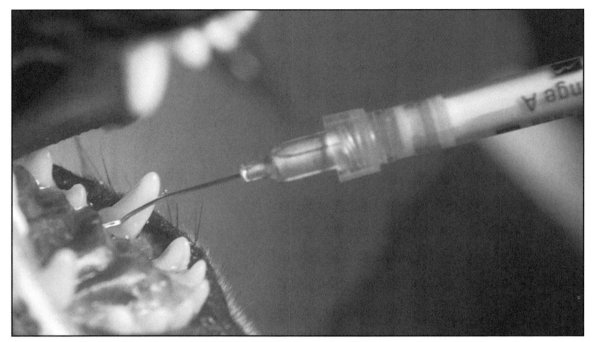

Figure 3.5 *Application of HESKA PERIOceutic GEL into the palatal pocket*

Starting a rigorous brushing program immediately following periodontal therapy is usually not recommended because of patient discomfort and the need to keep the perioceutics in place. Postoperatively using antimicrobial gels or solutions (chlorhexidine [CHX] or zinc—ascorbic acid products) is beneficial. Take care to follow the manufacturer's directions for certain products (e.g., Heska recommends that zinc products not be used and has provided some specific solutions to use).

Scheduling a recheck at 10 to 14 days can offer insight into potential complications and the anticipated outcome. Brushing can be started at this time. Schedule therapy in 4 to 6 months, depending on the extent of the problem.

Pockets up to 9 mm

Any pocket deeper than 5 mm must have adequate exposure for appropriate cleaning. Significant attachment loss is usually present in such lesions, so a full evaluation as to the viability of continued treatment is necessary.

Envelope Flap. Raise the gingival margin off the underlying bone with a periosteal elevator to expose the lesion. If no releasing incisions are made, the gingiva can be stretched if the gap is deep. The envelope should extend to at least one tooth on either side of the defect, and closure should be done with interdental sutures (absorbable 3-0 to 4-0 suture).

Releasing Flap. Make two releasing incisions to allow better exposure without stretching the gingiva excessively (Figure 3.6). Make these incisions one tooth away from the tooth to be treated and on a line approximately halfway between the midpoint of the root and the edge of the tooth (line angle). Do not make releasing lines in the interdental area, at the furcation (inter-radicular), or directly over the root. Excise a thin collarette of the free gingival margin to release the marginal flap and debride a narrow band of infected tissue but take care to preserve the maximum amount of attached gingiva. Release the flap just enough to expose the lesion without exposing an excessive amount of bone. For a full exposure of all tooth surfaces, you should elevate a palatal or lingual flap to visualize all potential lesions.

Simple closure returns the gingiva to its original height, with suturing done at the releasing incisions as well as at interdental spaces. For areas with horizontal bone loss, replace the gingiva farther down the root (*apical repositioning*), after releasing both facial and lingual flaps. Often, some alveolar recontouring is necessary to allow the gingiva to lie back down smoothly for suturing the interdental spaces.

Pedicle flaps and free gingival grafts to cover gingival defects are more advanced procedures that require additional knowledge and training, and they must be accompanied by meticulous home care and regular follow-ups.

Regenerative Therapy (Guided Tissue Regeneration, or GTR). Not too many years ago, it was believed that once periodontal tissues were lost, they were gone for good. Then, human dentistry began to explore therapy to stimulate the regrowth of healthy periodontal tissues, and veterinary dentistry has benefited greatly from the expertise that developed in this are.

The theory of regeneration focuses on allowing the correct cells to grow into the defect first—osteoblasts to recover bone loss and periodontal cells to bridge from bone to tooth. With the placement of some sort of barrier in the void, this

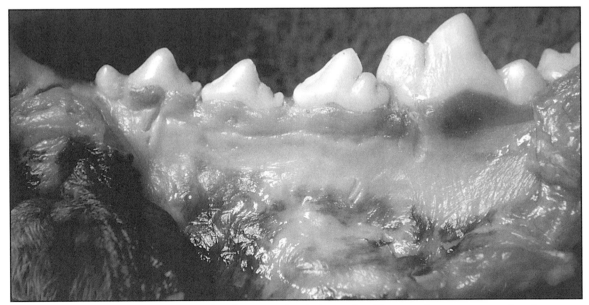

Figure 3.6 *Mesial and distal releasing incisions for flap and open-root planing*

therapy aims to keep the faster-growing alveolar mucosa and gingival connective tissue out of the defect, while encouraging growth of the periodontal ligament and bone.

Special barrier membranes are used extensively in human dentistry, modeled to protect specific types of defects. However, although membranes can be used in veterinary dentistry, bulk materials are generally easier to use and less expensive. Older references may describe the use of bulk materials such as tricalcium phosphate (TCP), calcium sulfate, and doxycycline. The calcium products provide a matrix for an organized clot and also provide calcium directly to the site; doxycycline can act both in an antibacterial capacity and as an anticollagenolytic agent. Once the bulk matter is in place, it should prevent the faster-growing soft-tissue cells from taking over the sulcus or pocket site. New osseopromotive products such as Consil (Nutramax, Baltimore, MD), a biosynthetic particulate glass material, optimally work both as a barrier and to stimulate new bone growth.

It is essential to adequately remove all debris and granulation tissue from the lesion in order to expose the alveolar walls and tooth surface lining the defect. Debridement to remove any necrotic debris and "freshen" the wound is also helpful. There also must be sufficient attached gingiva to protect the site and sufficient soft tissue with tension released to suture the site closed over the bulk material.

It is key to select the appropriate type of lesion for this therapy and use a proper technique. Ideally, you will have a specific site for bulk material placement, such as an infrabony pocket that is accessible by raising a gingival flap. A cup defect (four-walled) with a lesion located circumferentially around the tooth is sometimes difficult to adequately clean. Two- and three-walled interproximal defects and three-walled defects around single-rooted teeth are treatable sites. One-walled and some two-walled defects that have no support at one or more aspects of the defect will not retain materials as well. Depending on the extent of the lesion, some stage II furcational defects that do not pass all the way through to the other side of the tooth may also be treated. The relative importance of the tooth should also be taken into account: A significant pocket around the lower corner incisor may benefit more if the tooth is extracted in order to better preserve the adjacent canine. Certainly, the lower first molar is one of the most common sites for such bone loss, and regenerative therapy would definitely prove beneficial there. Use releasing incisions to open a gingival flap for exposure, and thoroughly debride the pocket, including any granulomatous tissue. Once the bulk material has been placed, suture the gingival flap closed.

Another site that could benefit from regenerative therapy is the palatal surface of the maxillary canine teeth. If left unchecked, bone loss at this site will eventually progress into an oronasal fistulation, necessitating extraction and fistula closure in most cases. If caught before such fistulation occurs, however, proper placement of the material can greatly enhance the chance of preserving the tooth and periodontium.

Access to the site can be a little tricky—a simple *envelope flap* won't move the palatal mucosa far enough out of the way for exposure. You can make mesial and distal incisions with elevation of the palatal mucosa, but again, the tissue is mainly just lifted higher and not necessarily moved out of the way in many cases. A crescent-shaped incision beginning near the mesial extent of the tooth and curving into the palate past the canine, with the flap elevated off the palate, will expose the defect (Figure 3.7; significant hemorrhaging can be expected— use digital pressure to minimize). Thorough debridement with curettes is essential prior to placing the osseogenic barrier material. Suture the flap mesially to fit snugly against the tooth and help secure and protect the material.

In defects in which an envelope flap or mesial and distal releasing incisions are sufficient, consider a sling suture pattern for the best closure. In this pattern, you will run the suture in the palatal submucosa in a half-circle pattern extending from the mesial to the distal aspect. You'll often have to exit the needle at approximately the halfway point, then reenter the tissue at the same site to continue the half-circle. Then reverse this path, running the suture in the half-circle from distal to mesial, close to the first pass, and exiting in the buccal mucosa close to the initial suture tail. When tied, this pattern pulls the flap tightly against the tooth without strangling tissue as a purse-string pattern would do.

With all procedures, a strong owner commitment is essential to maximize the prognosis. To keep postoperative tissue manipulation to a minimum, have the owners use oral rinses initially (chlorhexidine, zinc ascorbate), then start a brushing program after the first recheck 10 to 14 days later. Schedule follow-up treatment 3 to 4 months later, which should include reassessment with radiography and probing and possibly even retreatment.

Splinting Mobile Teeth. Mobility in teeth certainly decreases their chances for successful retention, and it is sometimes helpful to provide stability, particularly if the goal is osseous regeneration. Restorative products (composites, some reinforced) can be placed to bridge across teeth, with at least one stabile tooth present at each end. This is most frequently done with incisors, and meticulous home care is necessary to avoid any buildup of debris around the device. This method is not very effective in retaining a tooth that has minimal attachment with little chance of reattachment—it would just delay the inevitable.

HOME CARE

You may be able to provide the best professional dental care possible for your patients, but without a strong commitment from the owners to provide supportive care, the prognosis for the therapy will suffer. Certainly, an optimal level of home care is not attainable in all cases (in human dentistry, compliance rates are notoriously low), but with proper education and instruction, you can at least give pet owners the tools to try their best.

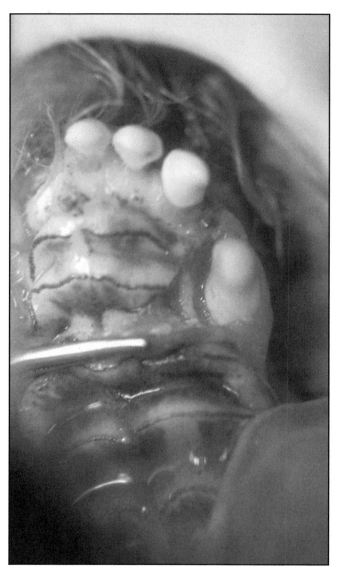

Figure 3.7a *Release of crescent flap to expose deep palatal pocket at a maxillary canine*

Client Education

To effectively convince clients of the benefits of good oral hygiene, you must first be convinced yourself. Whether providing information on home care for household animals or clinic "pets," both veterinarians and technicians must become more familiar and comfortable with the products available. Even being able to "spotlight" successful client-pet efforts due in part to home care can help show others that home care is not just a gimmick. You can use the clients' own level of personal oral care to guide them in seeing how beneficial care for their pets can be.

True, not every client (and especially not every pet) is going to be an ideal candidate for a rigorous home-care regimen. After all, you don't want to send clients to the emergency room every time they try to brush the teeth of an aggressive dog. Then, of course, there will be those who will laugh in your face at the suggestion that they brush their pets' teeth. But in many cases, the proper combination of training and technique can have positive results.

Brushing

Without a doubt, the mechanical process of brushing to physically remove soft deposits of plaque is the best way to provide adequate home care. All other products and methods strive to fight the bacteria in the plaque, but nothing compares to the tangible act of brushing.

Products

In the last few years, the number of brushing products on the market has increased exponentially. If a toothbrush will be used, select one that has soft bristles and is of an appropriate size for the pet's mouth. Pets should not share brushes, and toothbrushes should be replaced at regular intervals because of potential bacterial buildup in the bristles. Many sizes, shapes, and angles are available, from double-ended angled brushes to small cat brushes to soft children's toothbrushes.

For those pets who might be uncomfortable with a full brushing technique or during initial training, other devices can be used. Rubber finger cots with textured ends, gauze or rough-surfaced cloth finger wraps, and gauze pads can provide some abrasive action without the bulk of a brush.

Certainly, one consequence of the increased interest in dental products is the plethora of dentifrices available today. Sometimes, it is difficult to choose which one to use, and it is, of course, impossible to carry all the different brands for dispensing. The best plan of attack is to select a limited number of quality products (in all categories), with a choice of "flavors," and become familiar with those.

The one product to avoid is human toothpaste, which contains detergents for foaming and other ingredients, such as fluoride. These products are

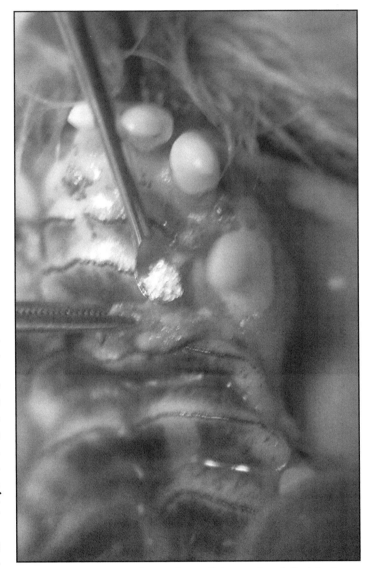

Figure 3.7b *Packing Consil into the debrided pocket*

fine for brushing if they are expectorated, but they can cause stomach irritation and even toxicity if ingested on a regular basis. Few dogs and cats know how to rinse and spit!

Some of the pet toothpastes may be enhanced with enzymatic activity that can inhibit the formation of plaque. Some contain low levels of fluoride for its antibacterial properties (caries are less of a concern in pets), but ingesting excessive amounts should be avoided.

Training

Ideally, some level of home care should be instituted when the pet is still young, but it is still possible to teach an old dog new tricks! The best way to approach home-care training is to start out slowly and progress gradually, which can be easier for pet and client alike.

For most animals and especially for those who might be head-shy, it is important to get them used to regular handling about the head and face. Training sessions should be brief initially, and a positive reinforcement should be given at the end. Slow, deliberate movements that are an extension of a caress help put the pet at ease. This can be particularly beneficial in cats, mimicking the action of head-rubbing or marking. Once the animal is comfortable with that, the owner can move the hand along the side of the mouth to gently pull the lips back, putting a little more direct pressure on the caudal teeth. If there is any concern about the animal accidentally nipping, the other hand can be used to hold the muzzle closed.

Rather than using a brush at first, use a gauze pad or thin washcloth to wipe the facial surfaces—especially of the incisors, canines, and upper fourth premolars. Water or flavored liquids (broth for dogs, the water in canned tuna for cats) can make the experience a little more pleasant at first, with progression to the flavored toothpastes later. Once the pet is comfortable with these actions, a soft-bristled brush can be introduced. Optimally, a brush is most effective when the bristles are aimed at a 45° angle into the sulcus and a circular brushing action is used (Figure 3.8). The rostral teeth (incisors and canines) and the maxillary premolars (buccal surfaces) are easiest to brush, but depending on the pet, brushing even the molars, mandibular teeth, and lingual surfaces is an attainable goal.

Oral Gels and Solutions

In some cases, full brushing is not an option either because of resistance to the effort or when brushing should be avoided immediately after periodontal surgery. There are also times where oral medicaments can be good adjunctive therapy to brushing and vice versa.

Chlorhexidine

The standard by which other oral products are often tested is chlorhexidine (usually tested in the gluconate form). As an antimicrobial that can bond to the *pellicle* layer on the tooth surface, chlorhexidine works against the primary building block of periodontal disease—bacteria. CHX seems to work best in the gluconate form, though CHX acetate products can also be effective. Optimal therapy keeps the CHX on the tooth surface for at least a minute, so the 0.2% solutions that humans rinse with may not be adequate in dogs and cats. More viscous gels allow the CHX to remain in contact with the tooth surface longer, and bioadhesive patches retained on the buccal mucosa can provide a more constant delivery.

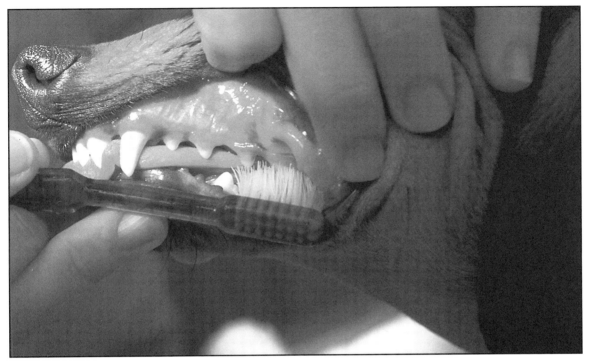

Figure 3.8 *Brushing*

Its bitter taste makes CHX difficult to use for home care even in diluted amounts, but it can sometimes be used as an irrigant during oral procedures. If any form of regenerative therapy is to be performed on a patient, avoid using CHX or at least rinse it well from the area because even low concentrations can be detrimental to periodontal cells.

Chronic use of CHX may stain the teeth, actually discoloring the *pellicle* as minerals are taken up by the product. Regular brushing when using CHX can minimize this effect.

Fluoride

As discussed earlier (as a step in the complete prophylaxis), you should use topical oral fluorides judiciously because of the potential for nephrotoxicity if excessive amounts are ingested. In addition, only fluorides that are effective in the presence of some moisture can be utilized as a home-care product. Stannous fluoride (0.4%) in glycerin is one of the more common forms used in veterinary medicine, with indications for use in teeth that have weakened or sensitive areas of enamel, as compared to caries prevention in man. Sodium fluoride (0.02%) is soluble in water and can be used in oral sprays, as can acidulated phosphate fluorides that may allow better penetration of the tooth surface given its acidity, thereby allowing remineralization with fluoride compounds.

Zinc Ascorbate

Zinc ascorbate gels or solutions can help in the short-term control of oral odor. In addition, zinc ascorbate's support of collagen synthesis and stimulation of healing are helpful traits in postsurgical cases.

Chewing Exercise

The primary purpose of teeth is to prehend and chew food, but quite often, other objects can be chewed on as well, with some pets being experts at this behavior! Chewing is certainly a necessary activity, but there are appropriate and inappropriate forms of chewing behavior and types of chewing materials. Many chew toys are purchased to satisfy a dog's chewing instincts, so the added benefit of plaque control for some is a plus. A wide range of devices are available, with a variety of possible effects. You should let owners know that even though these products might help with plaque control, they should be just a first step in a program that includes regular brushing, if at all possible.

On one hand, it takes the regular forces of mastication to keep the mouth healthy by using the musculature and stimulating compression of the periodontal ligament (even providing a natural cleansing of plaque off tooth surfaces, depending on the item[s] being chewed). Items that mimic the tooth chewing through a hide can provide some of the best plaque removal. Chewing devices that have more flexibility and "give," with a fibrous nature, are safer for the tooth as well. Rawhide strips, some of which have dentifrices in them, can provide good exercise. Larger, more solid rawhide toys should be checked carefully because a dog can break a tooth on these if enough force is used. Soaking such an item in water before giving it to the dog may make it a little more pliable. Harder chewing objects, such as cow hooves, bones, and compressed plastic items, may last longer, but the potential for tooth fracture is much greater, even with ice. You should closely monitor any dogs who are heavy chewers, paying attention especially to the carnassial teeth (upper fourth premolars, lower first molars). Always evaluate a fractured tooth for open canals or pulpal damage (see chapter 5: Advanced Oral and Dental Problems—Endodontics).

Though study results differ, a dry kibble diet generally gives a degree of abrasive action during chewing, which helps to wipe plaque and soft debris off some of the tooth surfaces. This action can be enhanced with specific diets and kibble designed not to crumble with the first chew. These morsels remain intact as the cusp enters them, providing a squeegee-type effect. Other diets may contain compounds that interfere with the mineralization of plaque into calculus.

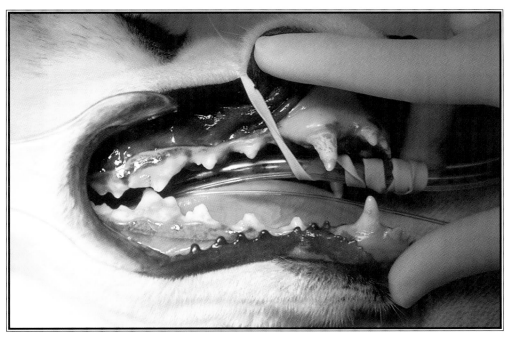

Plate 1 *Generalized enamel hypocalcification*

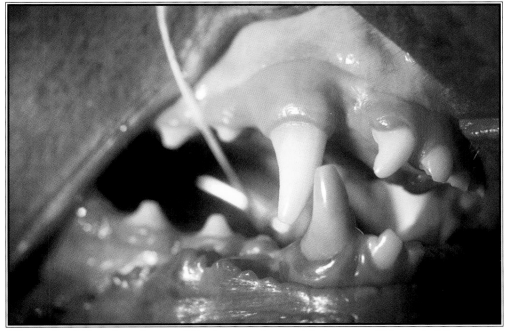

Plate 2—*Discolored mandibular canine, with irreversible pulpitis*

64

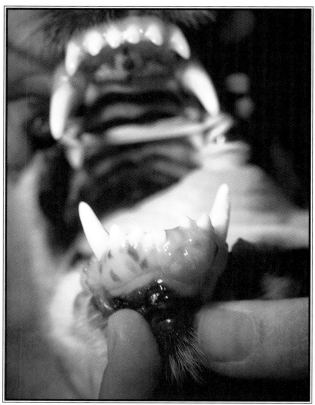

Plate 3 *Acanthomatous epulis of rostral mandible*

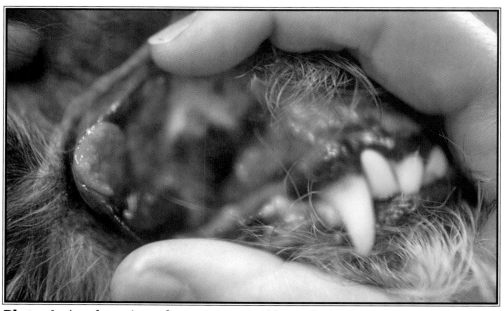

Plate 4 *Amelanotic melanosarcoma of buccal gingiva*

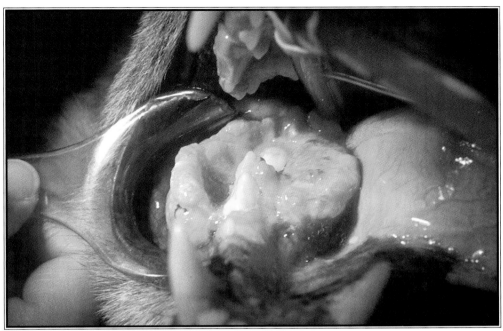

Plate 5 *Squamous cell carcinoma of canine mandible*

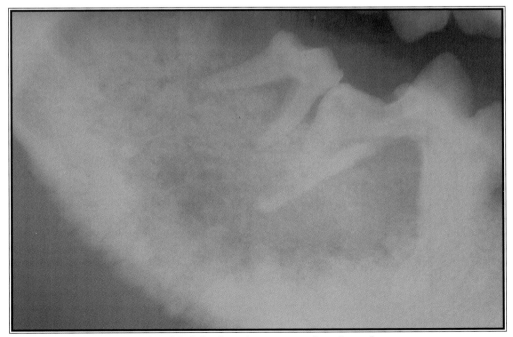

Plate 6 *Radiograph of SCC showing extension into bone*

66

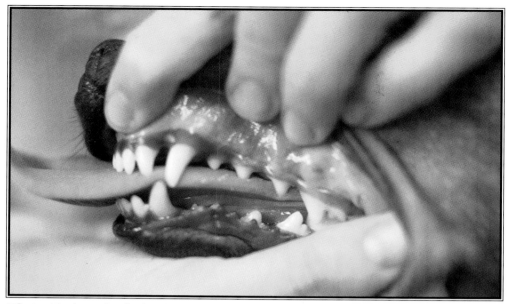

Plate 7 *Attached gingiva, separated at mucogingival line from alveolar mucosa*

Plate 8 *Chronic Ulcerative Paradental Stomatitis above a maxillary canine, no attached gingiva remaining*

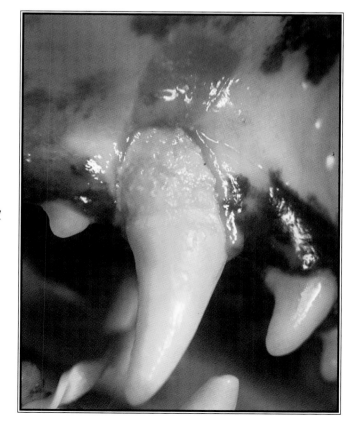

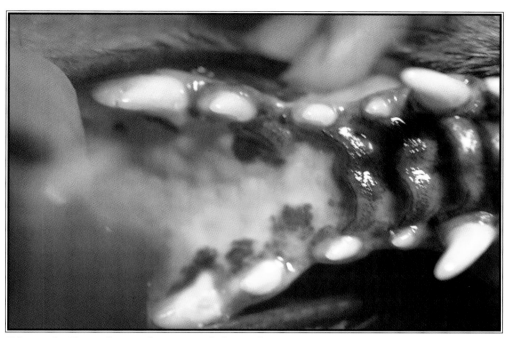

Plate 9 *Pemphigus lesions of the palate*

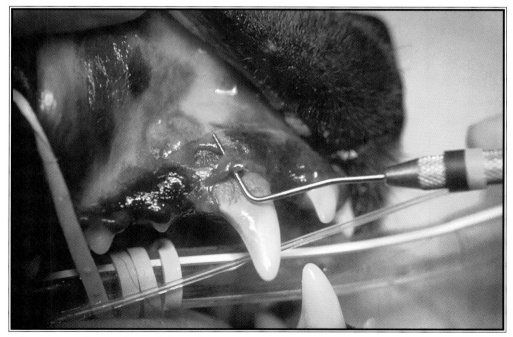

Plate 10 *Periodontal fistula at a maxillary canine*

68

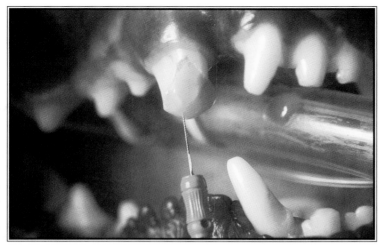

Plate 11 *Fractured maxillary canine tooth with pathfinder file in exposed canal (purulent)*

Plate 12 *Suborbital fistula from abscessed maxillary fourth premolar*

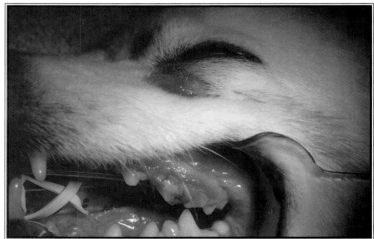

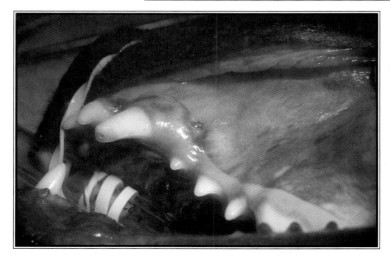

Plate 13 *Endodontic fistula in alveolar mucosa from abscessed maxillary cuspid*

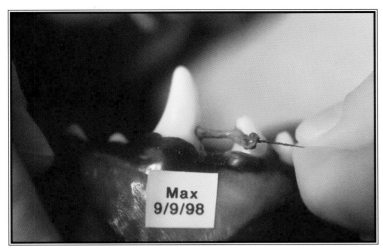

Plate 14 *Necrotic pulp removal from intact, nonvital tooth*

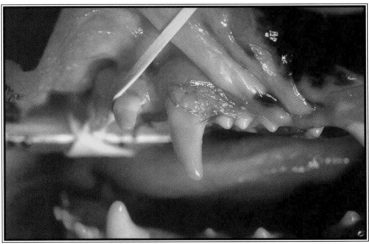

Plate 15
Damage caused by electrocautery treatment for gingival hyperplasia, nonvital teeth (discolored), necrotic alveolar bone

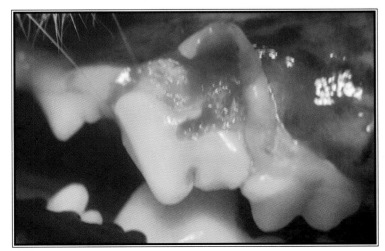

Plate 16
Resorptive lesion of canine maxillary fourth premolar

70

Plate 17
Stomatitis:
Ulcerative faucitis

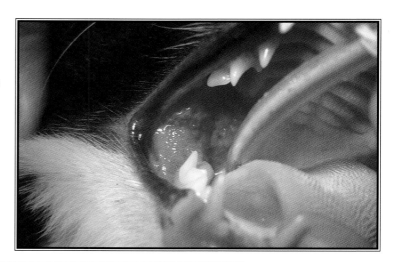

Plate 18
Stomatitis:
Proliferative
faucitis and
pharyngitis

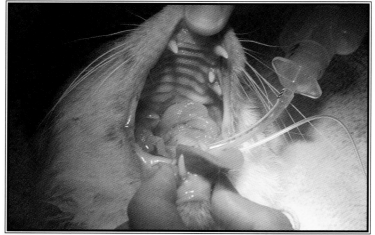

Plate 19
Stomatitis:
Sublingual
proliferation

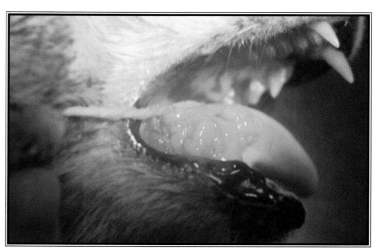

CHAPTER 4

Oral Surgery

Oral surgery incorporates many of the same basic principles and skills of both general soft-tissue surgery and osseous surgery. Wound management, suturing techniques, and even some aspects of fracture repair may be the same in the oral cavity as in other parts of the body. However, there are also some distinct differences that must be recognized if proper therapy is to be instituted.

PAIN MANAGEMENT

Certainly, one area that you should never overlook in any form of surgery is pain management. Thoroughly assessing the level of pain experienced by veterinary patients can be difficult given the great variation in individual responses to discomfort.

General Anesthesia

There are very few instances in oral surgery in which general anesthesia is not warranted. Take appropriate steps of preanesthetic screening as well as perioperative monitoring to minimize anesthetic risks for each patient. Specific anesthetic regimens will not be covered here, so you need to be fully aware of all aspects of your preferred protocol and the level of analgesia afforded. There is certainly validity in providing pain management prior to instigation of the procedure, before the stimulus is applied, not only for the patient's comfort but also to minimize the amount of general anesthesia needed for an adequate surgical plane. Using opioids as part of a preanesthetic regimen can enhance analgesic effect and help smooth induction and recovery.

Local Anesthesia

Adding a local anesthetic effect has benefits, particularly if it is administered before the procedure has started, to minimize the afferent stimulation. Various topical and injectable products are available, which should be chosen on the basis of their length of effectiveness and even the presence of epinephrine. Follow manufacturer's recommendations when appropriate, and pay attention to total doses used and any contraindications (e.g., the presence of heart disease in the patient or the use of halothane in combination with epinephrine).

ɔcal Infiltration

For smaller or focal areas, local infiltration of the injectable anesthesia can ɒe simply accomplished by injecting into the adjacent gingiva or mucosa or even into the periodontal ligament space for extractions.

Block Anesthesia

Specific areas can be used for anesthetic injection to affect a certain region of the oral cavity. Take care to focus on a particular area, as you might want to avoid extensive block anesthesia, especially for bilateral mandibular procedures, because the loss of feeling may lead to self-inflicted trauma from chewing of the cheeks or tongue.

Infraorbital Block. An anesthetic may be deposited at the rostral aspect of the infraorbital foramen located above the upper fourth premolar for analgesia in the rostral portion of the maxilla (Figure 4.1).

Deep Infraorbital Block. Place the needle deeper into the infraorbital foramen, using digital pressure at the rostral aspect of the foramen to force the injection into the canal. This can enhance the anesthetic effect to include more distal portions of the maxilla, including the upper fourth premolar. Carefully place the needle into the canal to keep the hub close to the bone and away from the nerves and vessels.

Mental Foramina Block. Local infiltration at the mental foramina will help to anesthetize the portion of mandible rostral to the site.

Caudal Mandibular (Mandibular Alveolar) Block. Inject the local at the medial aspect of the mandible at the entrance of the mandibular nerve into the mandibular canal to provide analgesia for a large portion of the mandible. The "notch" at the distoventral aspect of the mandible should be palpated, for it is a landmark for injection deposition. This block in particular should be done

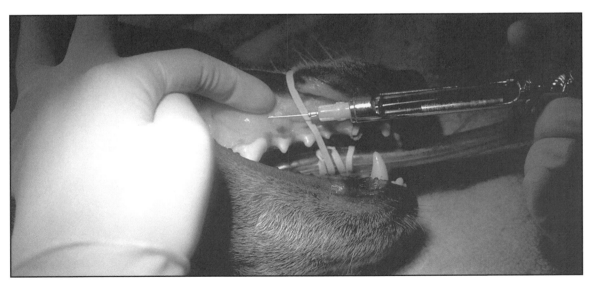

Figure 4.1 *Infraorbital block*

with great care bilaterally because of the potential injury the patient can inflict upon itself if the tissues remain numb for an extended period.

Postoperative Pain Management

Pain management postoperatively can be one of the most important aspects of the patient's care. If discomfort is going to result in self-traumatization of the surgical site, great damage can result. Providing sufficient comfort is also vital in returning the pet to adequate oral function, particularly in supporting the appetite in cats. Immediately after surgery, injectable analgesics (including opioids) can help to smooth the patient's recovery. The medication dispensed for home use can range from something as simple as buffered aspirin to butorphanol to fentanyl patches. Again, you will have to use products you are familiar with in order to individually customize the postsurgical instructions for each patient.

GENERAL SURGICAL POINTS

You make a number of critical decisions when approaching a surgical technique. Your decisions regarding appropriate procedure, suture material, and postoperative care can all influence the eventual outcome.

Suture Selection and Technique

There are certainly individual preferences as to what materials are chosen, but, in general, a reasonably small (3-0 to 4-0 or smaller), absorbable suture material, used with a reverse cutting needle, is best for most oral surgery. Your choices may vary according to the application of the suturing as well, from simple extractions in cats to major palatal reconstruction. Typically, a simple interrupted suture pattern is best used to appose oral tissues, though some techniques for minimizing tension (vertical mattress sutures) are also utilized.

Soft-Tissue Management

Because of some unusual stresses that can be encountered in the oral cavity (constant moisture, licking, respiratory pressures with oronasal fistulation), it is imperative that you close the site without any tension on the suture line. In addition, any portion of the epithelium that is incorporated into the suture line should not be intact but scarified or scraped to provide a healthy vascular bed for healing. Freshen intact gingival margins or chronic granulation beds before closure.

Osseous Management

Principles used in long-bone fixation for fracture repair can be extrapolated for use in the oral cavity, but it is imperative to maintain a functional occlusion, without sacrificing it for stability of the fracture site. Also, perform invasive fracture repair techniques only with great care because of the extensive damage that you can inflict on the roots or vascular canals (mandibular, suborbital).

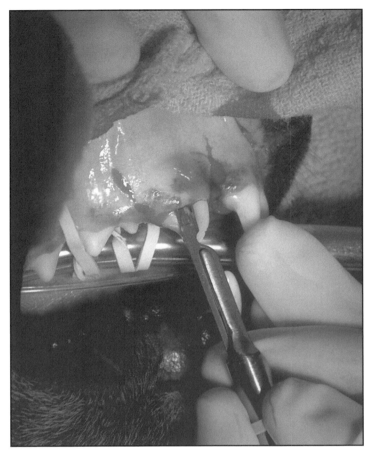

Figure 4.2 *Cutting the epithelial attachment between the two releasing incisions*

EXTRACTION

As a legal issue, it is imperative to have fully informed owner consent for an extraction before proceeding with any work. It is often difficult to predict if an extraction will be necessary at the time of the initial oral examination, so either obtain permission from the owner ahead of time or arrange for specific communication once the animal has been anesthetized and evaluated. If the owner has not given permission or cannot be located to approve a procedure, the procedure should not be done at that time.

Extraction Technique

Extractions can be very challenging, so a systematic approach is best in order to have consistent procedures and to minimize any unnecessary surprises. Trying to rush a procedure by bypassing simple steps can backfire, making things more difficult in the long run. Having good access and lighting and using the proper equipment (see chapter 9: Materials and Equipment) can make a big difference in the effort needed. The steps in a typical extraction procedure follow:

- Radiograph site
- Sever epithelial attachment
- Lift gingival flap
- Section roots
- Remove alveolar bone
- Luxate and elevate
- Elevate and extract
- Perform alveoloplasty and debridement
- Pack
- Suture

Radiograph Site

Both for accurate treatment planning and assessment and for complete medical records, it is essential to have good intraoral radiographs before and after extractions. Preoperative films can reveal a host of potential problems, including root resorption, fracture or *ankylosis,* supernumerary roots, and even dilacerated (curved) roots. They can also help distinguish deciduous teeth from permanent teeth and even reveal submerged supernumerary teeth. Post-operative films help to document complete root removal and the preservation of surrounding tissues (i.e., no fractures!).

Sever Epithelial Attachment

No matter how loose the tooth might be, if it is still attached to surrounding soft tissue, trying to remove it may damage the mucosa. Gently insert a small scalpel blade or periosteal elevator into the depth of the sulcus, and move it circumferentially around the tooth to cut the junctional epithelium or epithelial attachment.

Lift Gingival Flap

With most teeth, better access and visibility is beneficial, particularly when a gingival flap is raised. A simple envelope flap can stretch the gingival tissue, so you can use releasing incisions at the mesial and distal aspects of the tooth. Once you make the releasing incisions, cut the epithelial attachment (Figure 4.2) and elevate the gingival margin from the underlying bone by using the periosteal elevator. Advance the elevator from the gingival margin or from either releasing incision to gently separate the soft tissue without causing tears (Figure 4.3). Once you have released the flap to the level of the mucogingival junction, you can further minimize tension by gently excising the connecting fibers of the *periosteum* on the underside of the flap with small tissue scissors or the back of the scalpel blade (Figure 4.4). Place gentle traction on the flap while cutting the fibers to continue to raise the flap until it is adequately loosened. Having additional flexibility with the flap will allow adequate closure of the surgical site without any tension, even when closing across a gap, as with the upper fourth premolar or first molar.

Section Roots

You should divide all multirooted teeth into single-root components before making any attempt at elevation. Even loose teeth can have divergent roots that could be damaged with excessive extraction forces if not sectioned. Ideally, section the tooth from the furcation (easily visible with flap) toward the crown, with a crosscut bur on a high-speed handpiece with irrigation. Other methods may be necessary, including use of a *low-speed handpiece* (micromotor), with irrigation from a syringe or other water source, or even gigli wire passed through the furcation to cut up through the tooth. Avoid using cutting forceps to crack or break the tooth to avert potential complications of root and even jaw fracture.

Remove Alveolar Bone

You may need to remove some alveolar bone initially to expose the furcation adequately and, particularly in canine teeth and larger roots, both to expose the

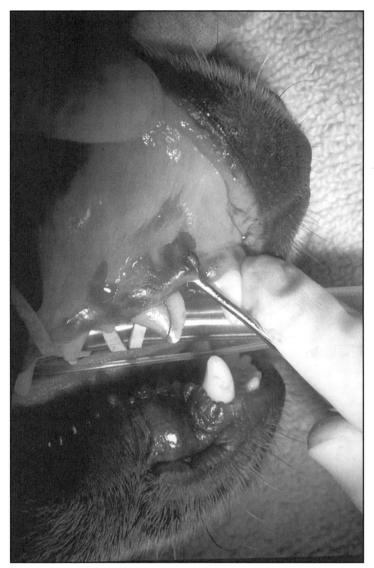

Figure 4.3 *Periosteal elevation of the flap*

widest part of the root and to create furrows into which you can place an elevator (Figure 4.5). If no progress is being made after the initial steps of elevation have been attempted, you can remove additional amounts of alveolar bone to facilitate the release of the root(s). With multirooted teeth, it may be best to remove more of the interradicular bone that is cancellous, as opposed to removing the stronger cortical alveolar bone plate, in order to preserve bone integrity. Additional amounts of alveolar plate may also need to be removed in order to adequately loosen up canine teeth as well.

Luxate and Elevate

The key to an ideal extraction of a relatively healthy tooth is to let the tissues work with you whenever possible. The periodontal ligament (PDL) holding the tooth to the alveolus is just that—a ligament that can be stretched and fatigued to the extent that the root can be loosened for easy removal. There are several methods of approaching the PDL, and often a number of methods are used on the same tooth. The primary goal is to provide sufficient gradual force to release the ligament's hold on the tooth without damaging any hard-tissue structure. Patience is definitely a virtue here.

Luxation. Introduce a luxator or elevator down into the periodontal ligament space along the root (Figure 4.6), with gradual pressure or rotation to press the root within the alveolus. PDL fibers can be stretched and torn, and you can even use the accompanying hemorrhage to advantage by allowing the pressure to fatigue the ligament further.

Leverage. You can also place the dental elevator between tooth sections, a section and adjacent tooth, or a section and adjacent bone. Several different methods of force can be applied, using the instrument as a lever against the fulcrum of the solid object. Once introduced, rotate or turn the elevator to engage the section with a moderate amount of pressure, and hold it steady in that position for 10 to 15 seconds (Figure 4.7). Use the elevator in different locations around a tooth, and with multiple sections or teeth, alternate the leverage from location to location to allow the hemorrhage in the periodontal ligament space to assist in fatiguing the ligament as well. Ideally, you should "elevate" the section straight out of the socket if the procedure has been performed correctly. Extraction forceps should not even be necessary, or if used, only minimal force should be required. Avoid the lateral or

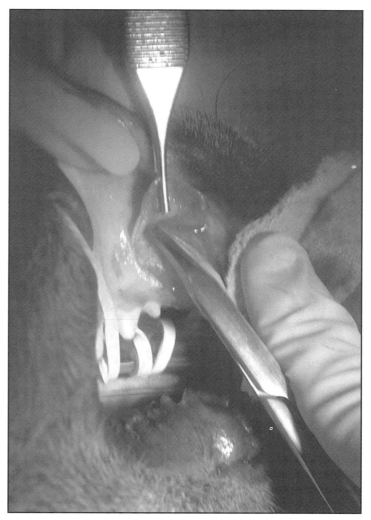

Figure 4.4 *Releasing the flap by excising attaching fibers*

labial elevation of the maxillary canine tooth crown because inadvertent medial deviation of the root could cause oronasal fistulation.

Elevate and Extract

Once you have sufficiently loosened the tooth section, the actual removal should be simple. At times, however, gentle pulling and rotating may be necessary to further loosen a tooth. Avoid excessive force, and if timely removal is not occurring, further elevation or alveolar bone removal may be necessary.

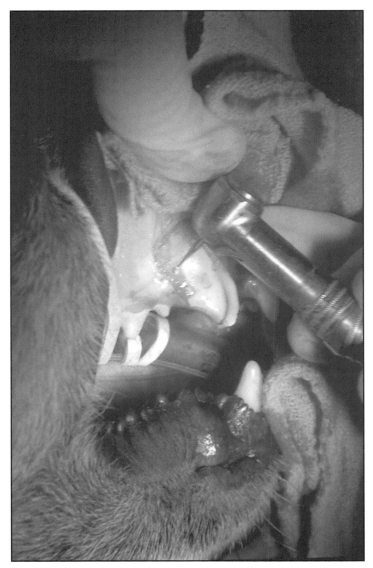

Figure 4.5 *Alveolar bone removal to expose root and make grooves for elevator placement*

Perform Alveoloplasty and Debridement

With the tooth section(s) removed, examine the alveolus for any damage. Curette and clean out any debris, and smooth or remove any sharp or roughened edges of alveolus (using a round bur on a high-speed handpiece or ronguers) (Figure 4.8).

Pack

In most cases, alveolar healing can be enhanced with the placement of an osseogenic material (Figure 4.9). Specific areas benefit greatly from use of such a product to help promote osseous healing, particularly where the bone integrity has been compromised. Extraction of mandibular first molars, especially when there has been periodontal bone loss, can endanger the strength of the mandible, so bone augmentation is definitely warranted. Maxillary canine alveoli, especially if periodontal bone loss has come close to causing an oronasal fistula, would also benefit from healthier bone, as can the rostral mandible with a mandibular canine removal that could compromise the area, particularly if bilateral extractions are done.

Suture

The most important concept in oral tissue closure is to avoid tension on the suture line at all costs. Releasing the flap contributes significantly to adequate closure, and, at times, you may need to extend the flap into the alveolar mucosa for sufficient laxity. It is best to have the suture line over solid bone, instead of a defect, and the close apposition of freshened epithelial margins enhances their healing capabilities. Scarify or roughen intact epithelial margins to provide a good vascular bed.

Specific Teeth

The anatomy of the tooth and even the surrounding structures may make some extractions challenging. If you follow specific steps when dealing with these difficult teeth, the extraction should proceed more smoothly.

Maxillary Canines

Make mesial and distal releasing incisions 1 to 2 mm from the actual tooth to have incisions closed over bone. A single releasing incision can sometimes provide sufficient access. You can be conservative with alveolar bone plate removal initially, removing a half-moon or u-shaped piece to expose the widest portion of the root and provide furrows in which to introduce the elevators. Additional plate removal may be necessary if the tooth does not start to loosen adequately. Avoid excessive elevation of the crown laterally (labially), as medial (palatal) displacement of the root could cause an oronasal fistula.

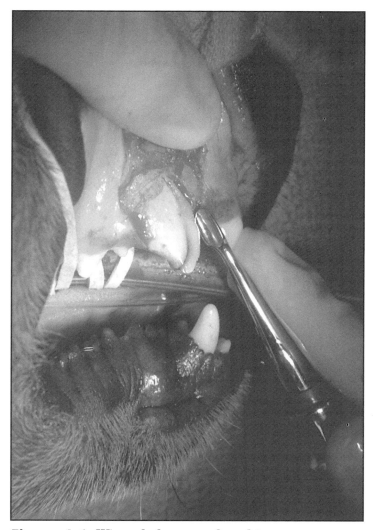

Figure 4.6 *Winged elevator placed into groove along root*

Mandibular Canines

Although there may be less alveolar bone mass on the lingual aspect of the tooth, important structures are present (sublingual vessels, nerves, salivary ducts). Labial plate removal is often sufficient. Take care not to elevate strenuously against the lower incisors, particularly if the mandibular symphysis is fibrous and mobile.

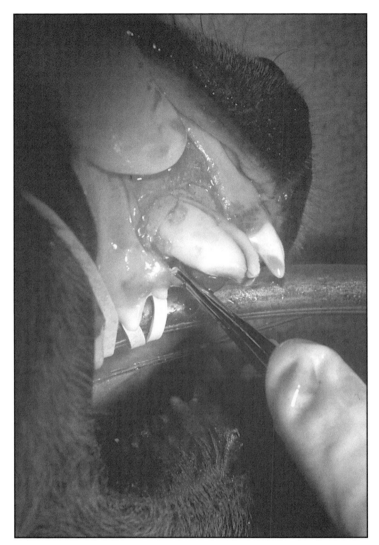

Figure 4.7 *Steady pressure with rotation to fatigue periodontal ligament*

Mandibular First Molars

It is imperative to radiograph these sites preoperatively to assess the integrity of the remaining mandibular bone. Sectioning the tooth is vital, and, at times, the larger mesial root will have a "retention groove" on its distal surface, making simple PDL fatigue difficult because of the lack of rotation. Promotion of osseous healing can help prevent a future mandibular fracture.

Deciduous Teeth

Deciduous teeth can be much more fragile and have very long roots in proportion to their crowns. In addition, perform any elevation attempts with great care to avoid damaging the permanent tooth bud if it hasn't yet erupted.

Feline Teeth

The small, delicate structure of some feline teeth can make their extraction more difficult, even when the difficulties encountered with resorption lesions and potentially ankylosed roots are not present. These teeth will be discussed more fully in chapter 7: Feline Oral and Dental Disease.

Complications

If you ignore the small details and steps of a systematic extraction, complications are more likely to occur. Using excessive force against tooth segments that are inadequately sectioned, exposed, or fatigued often leads to tooth or jaw fracture. Therefore, it is crucial that you be patient and take the time to complete all appropriate steps to avoid certain complications.

Broken Tooth or Roots

Given a choice, being able to extract the entire tooth segment with crown attached is definitely better than trying to dig out a root tip. If excessive force is used against the crown before the PDL has had a chance to loosen (or if the tooth is ankylosed), the fulcrum of the alveolar ridge can contribute to the tooth's fracture. Using extracting forceps to twist or pull the tooth before it is ready to come out is just asking for trouble. Once the root tip is broken, it can become very difficult to retrieve. Taking away additional alveolar bone (interradicular bone removal will leave more cortical bone), having good lighting, and using fine root-tip picks can help in retrieving the root fragment. Exercise care to not push the root tip further into the alveolus because if the apical extent of the alveolus is weak, the tip can be shoved into the mandibular canal or even the suborbital foramen, nasal cavity, or sinus. Once invulsed like that, root tips can be very difficult to remove, and extensive damage can be inflicted on the surrounding structures. Such root tips should be dislodged, however, to prevent a chronic foreign body reaction or infection.

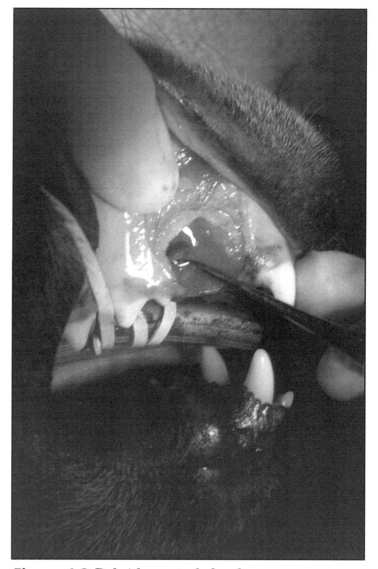

Figure 4.8 *Debridement of alveolus*

Ankylosed and Resorbing Roots

Retrieval of ankylosed root tips can be nearly impossible at times, as osseous changes may have already occurred. Seldom should you leave roots, and you should make every reasonable attempt to extract all tooth structure,

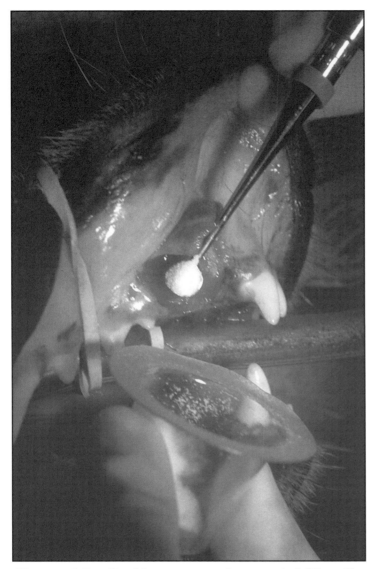

Figure 4.9a *Packing osseogenic material (Consil) into alveolus*

particularly if there is concurrent infection in the area, or if stomatitis is present. If partial removal is completely unavoidable, thorough records should be kept, and the owner should be made aware of the situation and given the recommendation to have the area radiographed in the future to monitor for any complications.

Pulverization is not the best method for root removal, but if attempted, it must be accompanied by intraoral radiographs to accurately assess the procedure. Good visual exposure can also be very helpful. Improper technique and inadequate irrigation can cause more harm than good.

Jaw Fracture

Though any area of the oral cavity can be traumatized with improper extraction forces, iatrogenic fracture probably occurs most frequently in the region of the mandible near the first molar. Particularly when there has been significant bone loss around one or both of the roots as a result of periodontal disease, substantial amounts of solid alveolar bone loss can greatly compromise the jaw strength (Figure 4.10). Thus, you must take great care in your preoperative assessment (radiograph) and surgical technique to minimize the likelihood of fracture. Certainly, full gingival flaps and tooth sectioning are vital, but steady and gradual forces of elevation, while properly supporting the mandible with the opposite hand, can ease the process. Postoperative radiographs provide good evidence of proper procedure. This is one site where *alveolar ridge* augmentation with osseogenic materials is advisable to avoid a future fracture in the region.

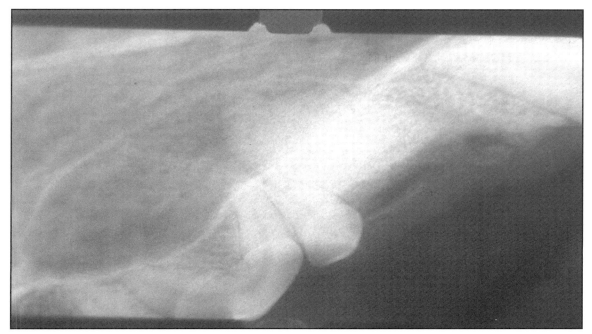

Figure 4.9b *Radiograph showing material in alveolus*

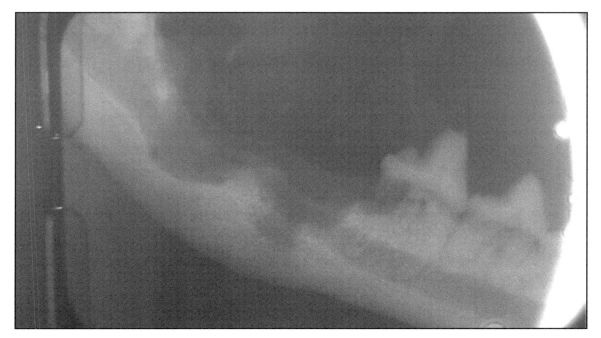

Figure 4.10 *Compromised mandibular bone at site of first molar periodontal disease postextraction*

Perforation

When correctly held with a finger guiding the shaft of the working head of the elevator, slipping shouldn't occur, but lax instrument control is a common cause for the perforation of structures around alveoli. The most damage can be done during extraction of the upper fourth premolar or first molar because of the proximity of the orbital cavity and suborbital canal structures (vessels, nerves). The mandibular canal can also be damaged with improper technique, and sublingual structures are susceptible to accidents as well.

Oronasal Fistula

Aggressive elevation on the palatal aspect of the maxillary canines can cause the instrument to perforate into the nasal cavity, particularly if the bone is already compromised. In addition, leverage of the crown laterally can cause the root to move palatally, even through the bone plate.

ORONASAL FISTULATION

Whether the loss of bone integrity between the maxillary canine and nasal cavity was caused by iatrogenic or other means (periodontal), the net effect is still the same. Similar defects can be caused in premolars, particularly the upper fourth, with communication into the nasal sinus (oroantral fistula). The opening, no matter how small, provides a constant pathway to introduce oral bacteria and debris into the nasal cavity, often causing chronic infection. It is imperative to be able to close the fistulation, and extraction (if the tooth is not already lost) should be followed by a specific flap procedure to help close this particular site. Even if you use meticulous technique, inform the owner that the persistence of a small opening is not unusual and that the patient will therefore have to be monitored and might need additional surgery in the future, though it should be relatively minor.

Mucoperiosteal Flap

You can use the simple or single mucoperiosteal flap if the fistula is recent and there has not been excessive structural loss of attached gingiva and buccal alveolar bone.

Procedure

If the tooth is still present, the standard extraction steps of making the mesial and distal releasing incisions and excising the gingival margin to provide a fresh edge should precede actual elevation. Preservation of the maximum amount of alveolar bone is important, as long as you can safely elevate the tooth.

If the tooth has already been lost, first excise or debride the edges of the opening by removing a collarette of the buccal gingival margin and by scarifying any intact epithelium at the palatal aspect. If the fistula is an extension of a deep palatal pocket, gently debride the area. Make releasing incisions at the mesial and distal aspects of the lesion past the level of the mucogingival junction (see Figure 4.2). You can make these incisions 2 to 3 mm out from the defect to provide a healthy osseous shelf to support the suture line. These incisions should diverge slightly to provide a wide base and enhance vascular supply. Use a periosteal elevator (Molt #2 or #4) to elevate the flap, preferably including the periosteum. Carefully advance the flat spoon shape of the periosteal elevator under the flap between it and the bone or even from the sides, starting at the releasing incisions, to a level just past the mucogingival junction.

Probably the most important concept to master in regard to flap preparation is to release the flap by excising the periosteal attachment on the underside of the flap (see Figure 4.4). Use the back end of a scalpel blade or small, sharp scissors to cut the fibers as you gently lift the flap, without going through the flap. The amount of release this provides can be significant and is extremely vital in minimizing tension on the flap.

Once sufficient release is attained, suture the flap to the opposite side of the deficit with simple interrupted sutures of 3-0 to 5-0 absorbable material. Place the sutures 1 to 2 mm apart, starting at one corner and working toward the other corner, with no gaps and absolutely no tension.

Postoperative Care

Instruct the owners to minimize handling of the area (lifting up the lip) postoperatively to avoid undue stress on the suture line. Schedule rechecks to monitor for any partial dehiscence, which can be expected at times. Such persistent openings are typically minor and can be repaired easily on a subsequent visit.

Double Flap

If the oronasal fistula has been chronic in nature or if significant amounts of associated tissue have been lost, a more advanced, double-flap procedure may be necessary to harvest material from the palatal mucosa to adequately cover the site. You may also need to use this procedure if previous, unsuccessful attempts at simple closure have resulted in fibrous scar tissue.

Procedure

Planning is an important first step in this procedure. Often, the palatal flap must extend to the midline or beyond it to provide sufficient coverage. If your patient has bilateral oronasal fistulations (ONFs), you must decide which side would benefit most from the palatal flap or, conversely, which side would respond best to a single mucoperiosteal flap. Using a surgical marker, you should outline the planned flap. The buccal flap should also be marked at this time, whether it is a mucoperiosteal flap or a finger-shaped pedicle flap. The pedicle flap consists of a distal or caudal base preserved in the alveolar mucosa above the distal extent of the defect with two parallel incisions extending rostrally. You should make this flap one and one-half times the width of the defect to allow for shrinkage and as long as necessary to cover the defect and the site of the palatal flap harvest site, once rotated. The flap is harvested from the buccal alveolar mucosa and elevated gently, preserving underlying structures (nerves, vessels, etc.).

The palatal flap's mesial and distal incisions should allow for a flap slightly wider than the original defect, to permit debridement of the defect edges and to preferentially place the suture lines over bone. Depending on the thickness of the flap (split thickness preserves some palatal bone, but full thickness provides a stronger flap), you can attempt to incorporate the palatine artery at the distal aspect of the flap. If cut, ligate it if possible, but be prepared for significant hemorrhage that may occur with such a procedure. These two incisions are joined by a third incision near or past the midline, depending on the extent of the defect. The margin of the defect associated with the flap must remain intact.

Elevate and lift the flap by using small, sharp scissors and a periosteal elevator, until sufficient release is attained to invert the flap back over on itself and the defect, still attached on the fourth side, so the palatal mucosa is now facing the nasal cavity. Debride the remaining three sides of the defect that are to receive the flap, retaining some tissue at the buccal aspect for suturing but scarifying any intact epithelial edges.

Suture the palatal flap in place securely with simple interrupted sutures, placed without gaps. Rotate the pedicle flap 90° to extend over the inverted palatal flap and its harvest site, suturing it in place. Close the defect caused by raising the pedicle flap by suturing the cut edges in apposition. Instead of using a pedicle flap, you can harvest a mucoperiosteal flap to cover the initial flap, though it's typically more difficult to extend it far enough to cover the palatal harvest site. Postoperative care is similar to that of the simple flap.

GINGIVAL HYPERPLASIA

With certain individuals, particularly boxers, gingival response to inflammation can result in hyperplastic tissue, sometimes excessive enough to cover the teeth (Figure 4.11). Such tissue results in increased pocket depth, even though the level of attachment remains the same, forming pseudopockets caused by excessive gingival height alone. Because the amount of attached gingiva is increased, therapy consists of excising the excess tissue to reduce pocket depths to a more normal level.

Assessment

You can mark the extent of the hyperplasia by measuring the pocket depth with a periodontal probe and indicating this depth on the outside of the gingiva by pressing the tip into the tissue at the measured level. This creates a bleeding point that you can repeat at regular intervals to outline the attachment level.

Excision

Using the bleeding points as a guide, you can use several methods of excision. With generalized hyperplasia, it is primarily an exercise in perseverance. Initially use sharp scissors with short, strong blades to debulk larger areas of tissues, particularly when pedunculated. Scalpel blades can connect the

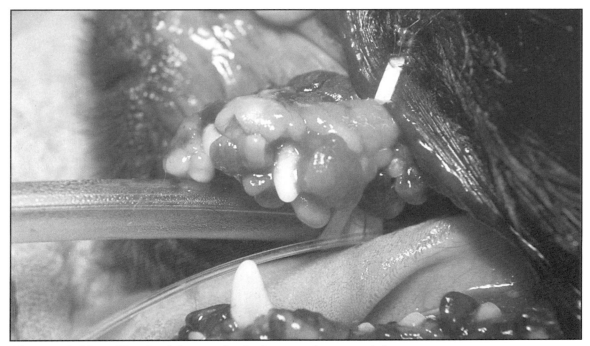

Figure 4.11a *Gingival hyperplasia in a cocker spaniel*

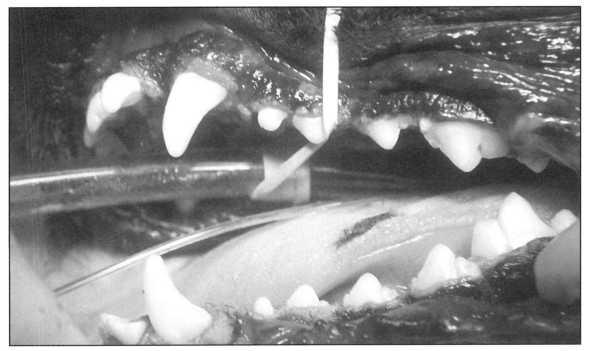

Figure 4.11b *Postoperative appearance*

bleeding point and form a scalloped, feathered gingival edge, but the blades need to be replaced on a regular basis when the gingival cutting dulls them. Electrosurgery (*partially* to *fully rectified current*) can also produce a sculpted margin with better hemorrhage control. With this method, you must use extreme care to avoid hyperthermic damage to the teeth and alveolar bone. Twelve-fluted burs on a high-speed handpiece with water for cooling can be used to provide a contoured margin as well. Submit any abnormal-looking tissue for histopathology.

Control hemorrhage with gentle pressure, moderate use of local anesthetics with dilute epinephrine (if indicated), and topical agents. Tincture of myrrh and benzoin can be used as gingival dressing to soothe the tissue.

Postoperative Care

Instruct the owners to gently apply oral rinses or gels (zinc ascorbate, chlorhexidine) initially, with regular brushing to begin at 10 to 14 days, depending on the patient's comfort level. Moderate levels of pain relievers may be needed if there is significant postoperative discomfort. Recurrence of the condition is not uncommon, but good oral hygiene may slow it.

EPULIS REMOVAL

An epulis may initially appear as a focal form of gingival hyperplasia, but because it arises from the periodontal ligament, surface excision is insufficient. Submit any abnormal-looking tissue for histopathological examination.

Extraction with Excision

For fibrous and ossifying epulides, complete excision of the mass must be combined with extraction of the tooth and curettage of the alveolus to debride the periodontal ligament. Without complete removal of the PDL, the mass can recur. Moderate en bloc resection that will effectively remove the PDL is also adequate.

En Bloc Removal

With a locally invasive acanthomatous epulis, surgical excision must be more aggressive. En bloc resection with clean margins can sometimes entail more advanced surgical techniques, such as rostral mandibulectomy or segmental resection. Such techniques are also used for resection of oral malignancies, but they are beyond the scope of this text. (See References and Recommended Readings at end of book.)

MISCELLANEOUS SOFT-TISSUE SURGERY

There are many indications for oral soft-tissue surgery, from gingival laceration repair to palatal reconstruction. Some of these are covered in chapter 6: Oral and Dental Emergencies (especially the sections on lip avulsion, gingival tears, etc.), and others are covered so extensively in general surgical and dental texts that we defer to those references (regarding palatal surgery, facial reconstruction, etc.). A few simpler procedures that might be indicated when specific oral abnormalities are encountered are covered here.

Tight Lip (Chinese Shar Pei)

In this condition, in which the bottom lip curls up and over the mandibular incisors and even canines, the actual defect is a diminished vestibular space of the rostral mandibular lip. Repair with an external stay suture in young dogs with a mild condition may be helpful, but often the vestibular depth itself needs correction. Simple excision with blunt dissection to open the space would not work as the nonepithelialized surfaces would heal back together quickly. A section of Penrose drain, cut open lengthwise and trimmed to fit the elliptical lesion, can be sutured to the surfaces until they epithelialize. Another method is to take the u-shaped (cross-section) layer of vestibular epithelium, release it just below the mucocutaneous level of the lip, elevate the layer, open the *vestibule* depth with blunt dissection, and use the layer to "line" the vestibule on the side of the mandible. In addition, you can harvest the periosteum from the rostral mandible to suture to the interior layer of the lip (Figure 4.12).

Frenectomy

In addition to vestibular deepening, releasing the tension the bilateral frenula place in the region may also be helpful. Make a rostral-to-caudal (mesial-to-distal) incision in both frenula halfway from where they attach close to the lower canines. Place the first interrupted suture to appose the mesial and distal aspects of the incision in a transverse closure. You may also use this procedure to relieve tension in cases with periodontal disease at the distal aspect of the mandibular canines.

Cheiloplasty

Cheiloplasty often involves additional closure of the lips in pets with redundant lips that tend to pool saliva and cause chronic irritation and infection or as an adjunct therapy with mandibulectomies to help keep the tongue inside the mouth. The most common procedure involves excising the area surrounding the mucocutaneous region on the caudal upper and lower lips. Use a two-layer closure (oral mucosa to oral mucosa or skin to skin) to appose the tissues. Apply a muzzle or tape the muzzle postoperatively to prevent excessive mouth opening until the site is healed.

Figure 4.12a *Tight-lip syndrome*

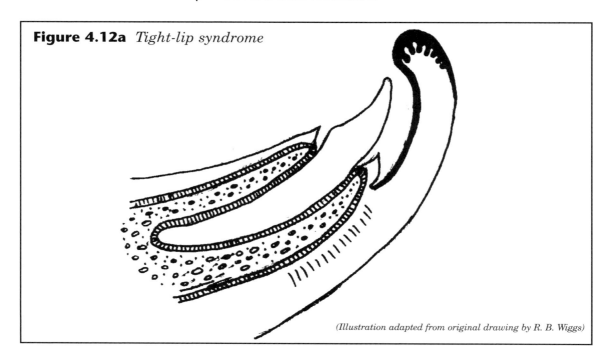

(Illustration adapted from original drawing by R. B. Wiggs)

Figure 4.12b *Incision to release buccal mucosa below mucocutaneous junction of lip*

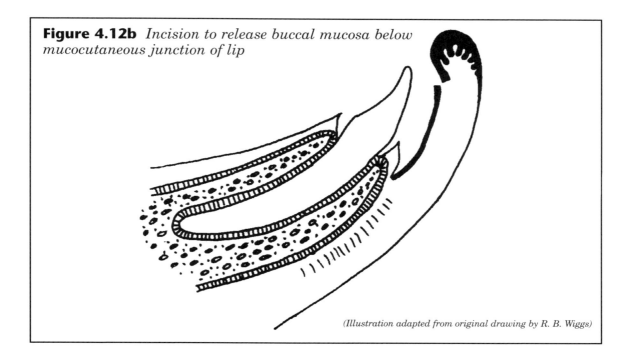

(Illustration adapted from original drawing by R. B. Wiggs)

Figure 4.12c *Release of buccal mucosa flap (dark); elevation of periosteal flap (lined) from ventral mandible*

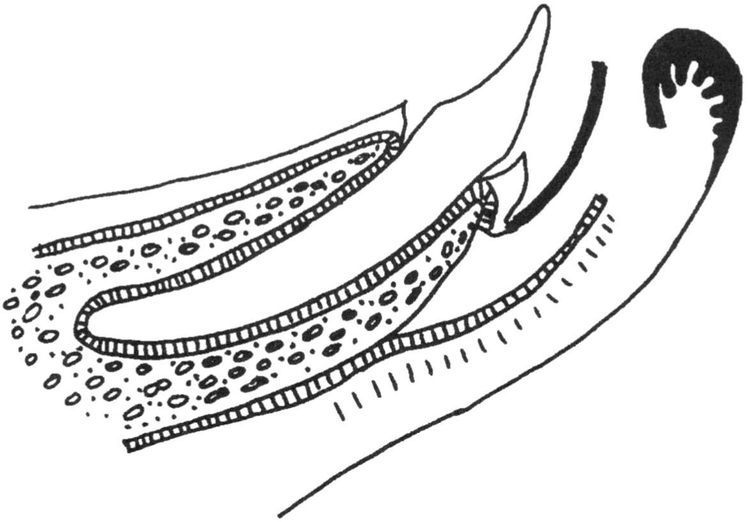

(Illustration adapted from original drawing by R. B. Wiggs)

Figure 4.12d *Placement of buccal mucosal flap (dark) against mandible, to be sutured into the depth of the vestibule; placement of periosteal flap (lined) to cover*
buccal harvest site

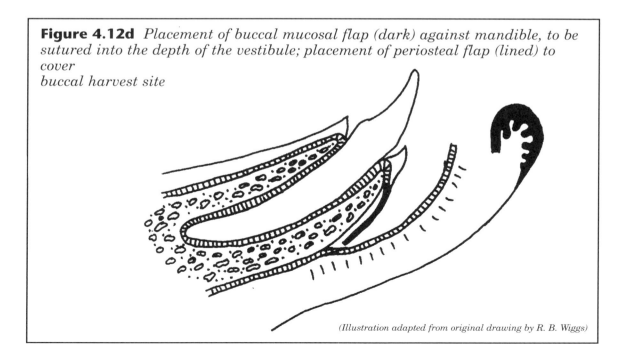

(Illustration adapted from original drawing by R. B. Wiggs)

Figure 4.12e *Flaps sutured in place; vestibular vault deepened*

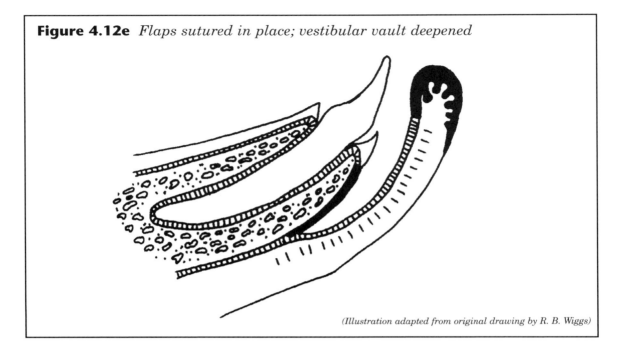

(Illustration adapted from original drawing by R. B. Wiggs)

CHAPTER 5

Advanced Oral and Dental Problems

Basic dental skills will not suffice for all of the oral and dental pathology you may encounter. However, you need to be able to recognize any abnormality and understand what therapy options are available, including possibilities of referral or alternative treatments. Of all the therapies described in this chapter, most require advanced knowledge and skills. The one situation that would warrant some attempt at treatment would be a recently exposed pulp. In this, time is of the essence for the prognosis, so if you can offer even a chance of saving the pulp, you should attempt to do so. If the procedure is not successful and the pulp eventually dies (and even the best-performed procedures can fail), other options, such as standard endodontics or extraction, are still possible.

ENDODONTICS

Outside of periodontics, problems involving the pulp canal system are probably the second most common type in veterinary dentistry. Many times, however, patients may give no indication that their broken or discolored teeth are even bothering them, until a more dramatic sign such as a suborbital fistula occurs. Nonetheless, anytime a tooth's endodontic system is compromised, it needs treatment.

Pulp Canal Exposure

Because the pulp canal is typically a closed, protected system outside of the apical communication, any breach can be detrimental. The most common means of canal exposure is tooth fracture (Plate 11), sometimes caused by external trauma, but in dogs it is frequently caused by chewing hard objects, such as cow hooves, bones, ice, rocks, and even hard chew toys. More gradual wear, again often from attrition (even from chewing on hair in cases of dermatitis), may be moderate enough to allow the odontoblasts of the pulp to provide a "retreat" for the pulp, producing dentin in the coronal portions that protects the pulp as the canal height diminishes. This reparative dentin will be brown to dark-brown in the center, feel smooth as you run the explorer across the top, and have no apparent canal opening. As long as the dentin is placed down faster than the tooth is worn away, the pulp remains protected. Attrition that debrides the tooth structure away faster than the dentin can be formed, however, will lead to pulp exposure, which appears as a black center with an open canal.

The process of bacterial decay in carious lesions can certainly lead to canal exposure, particularly once the decay reaches the dentin, where it can progress rapidly. The areas most commonly affected are the occlusal surfaces of the upper first molars and lower molars in the dog. Typically, the lesion is too far advanced for salvage when detected, but if caught early, it may be treatable.

The pulp can sometimes be left unprotected as well by developmental abnormalities. Changes may range from a disruption in the hard-tissue deposition (enamel and cementum) to an infolding of the enamel into the tooth structure (dens-in-dente). Any exposure of the pulp can lead to its infection and its death.

Once the canal is open, it is exposed to bacteria, and the pulp is infected. If left untreated, the pulp will die, and the infection will extend through the apex to involve the alveolar bone around the root. This can lead to periapical bone loss, apparent radiographically as a halo around the apex, caused by the formation of either a granuloma or an abscess that could eventually fistulate. A fistula will generally be past the mucogingival line, in the buccal mucosa, or it can extend externally in the suborbital region (upper fourth premolar) or ventral mandible (lower canine or first molar) (Plates 12 and 13). At times, a periapical infection can extend up the root to involve the entire periodontal attachment of the tooth or root, causing an endodontic-periodontic lesion or a combined perio-endo lesion if periodontal attachment loss is concurrently present.

Pulpitis

Even without apparent external structural damage that can expose the canal, the pulpal tissue itself can be compromised by a variety of stimuli. The blunt trauma of chewing hard objects that can fracture teeth can also cause enough occlusal pressure that the pulp can become inflamed and experience hemorrhage, even with a closed canal. This initial pulpitis will appear as a pink tooth due to the blood pigments seeping into the dentinal tubules. Pulpitis can be reversible, particularly in younger animals with wide canals and good blood supply. If the inflammation is severe enough, however, the edema can cause the death and necrosis of the pulp, in which case the tooth will turn a purple to gray color as the pigments in the tubules deteriorate.

Though not exposed to the external environment, a nonvital pulp can become infected due to the anachoretic introduction of bacteria from the systemic circulation into the apical blood supply. From that point, the infection can progress as described earlier, then extend into the periapical tissues and back into the systemic bloodstream. When such teeth are opened for endodontic access, the contents are sometimes necrotic (Plate 14).

Other stimuli that can injure a pulp include hyperthermia, often from iatrogenic sources such as the inappropriate use of ultrasonic scalers, prophy angles, and electrocautery (Plate 15). Electrical current from chewing on power cords can also damage the pulp, as well as gingival tissue and alveolar bone, in addition to causing systemic problems.

Treatment Options

Obviously, even if such an infection is not detectable and even if the pet shows no sign of discomfort, the condition should never be ignored! A nonvital pulp provides a bacterial "superhighway" that can continually introduce pathogens into the bloodstream, potentially affecting other systemic organs. This infection can progress subclinically for long periods of time undetected, so it is vital never to overlook a tooth with an endodontically compromised pulp.

Recent Canal Exposure

When a tooth fracture has opened the canal, the entire pulp does not die immediately. If the infected portion of the pulp can be removed before the rest of the pulp is affected and if it is treated appropriately, the remaining pulp has a chance to retain its viability (vital *pulpotomy*).

Timing of Therapy. In young animals (18 months of age) with a wide canal and good blood supply, you can attempt the vital pulpotomy procedure up to 2 weeks after canal exposure. Keeping the pulp functional is beneficial in this age group to allow continued tooth maturation (thicker dentinal walls, apex closure). In fact, in an immature permanent tooth with an open apex, this attempt should be made if at all possible.

With patients older than 18 months of age, the window of opportunity is narrowed to about 5 days after the fracture. Unless you can treat the pulp within this period after canal exposure, the likelihood of it becoming nonvital increases.

Medical Support. To minimize the risk of infection and inflammation immediately after tooth fracture and after the pulpotomy procedure, you can recommend antibiotics and anti-inflammatory agents. Take care with non-steroidal anti-inflammatory drugs (NSAIDs) or other compounds that might affect platelets or clotting because hemorrhage control is an important step in the therapy.

Vital Pulpotomy and Pulp Capping. With a recent canal exposure, you should first try to clean and isolate the area (using chlorhexidine and a dental dam). Take a radiograph to evaluate tooth maturity, apical pathology, and root integrity. Remove the coronal portion of the pulp tissue down to about the level of the cervical region or neck of the tooth (approximately 5 mm), using a round bur (high-speed handpiece with water) or an endodontic spoon. This should remove the inflamed pulp down to a level of healthy tissue. If this is the case, you should be able to control any hemorrhaging with relative ease, generally within 5 minutes. Place the blunt end of sterile paper points into the canal to absorb free blood and encourage coagulation. Soak a paper point in small amounts of lidocaine with epinephrine, and introduce it into the canal for additional hemorrhage control. Some nasal sprays applied to the pulp on a paper point can also temporarily help with the bleeding. If bleeding is persistent, it may be an indication that the pulp was more inflamed than initially thought, and you may need to remove additional amounts of pulp to reach healthy tissue, if any remains.

Figure 5.1 *Vital pulpotomy*

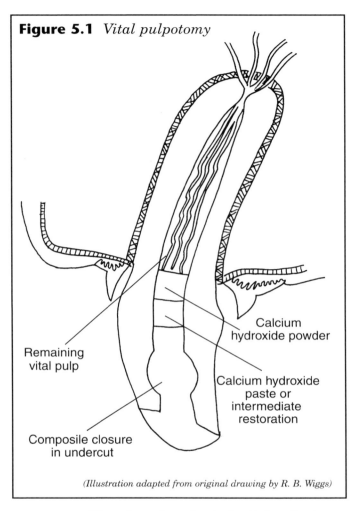

Remaining
vital pulp

Calcium
hydroxide powder

Calcium hydroxide
paste or
intermediate
restoration

Composile closure
in undercut

(Illustration adapted from original drawing by R. B. Wiggs)

Next, place a layer of calcium hydroxide powder on top of the pulp using the moistened end of a paper point or retrograde amalgam carrier, and pack it down gently (in a 1-mm layer). This calcium hydroxide actually irritates the pulp, stimulating it to form a reparative dentinal bridge that will protect the pulp at that level. Then place a layer of calcium hydroxide paste on top of the calcium hydroxide powder or use a glass ionomer for a better seal. Finish with a composite closure. Radiograph immediately postoperatively, including a view of the opposing tooth. This will be used to compare to future radiographs (at 6 and 12 months) to confirm the success of the procedure (dentin walls continue to thicken, canal space narrows). Given the many variables involved, including the technique's sensitivity, residual pulp inflammation, and the questionable viability of the pulp, some procedures can be expected to fail (around 20%). If the tooth does become nonvital, other options may be necessary.

The steps in a typical vital pulpotomy and pulp capping procedure follow (see Figure 5.1):

- Clean and isolate area
- Radiograph site
- Remove coronal pulp
- Control hemorrhage
- Apply calcium hydroxide powder or paste
- Apply intermediate restorative (glass ionomer)
- Apply restorative
- Follow up

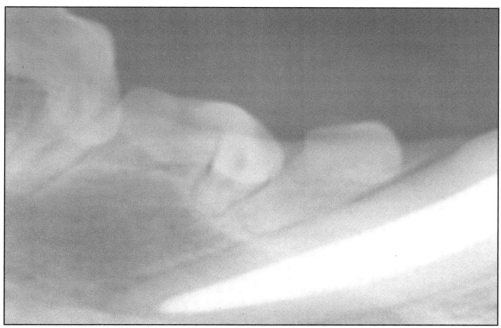

Figure 5.2 *Endodontic fill of mandibular canine (wide canal)*

Nonvital Pulp

Once a pulp becomes nonvital or compromised sufficiently so that it would probably not survive, it generally needs to be removed.

Standard Endodontics. If the tooth is mature with a closed, solid apex, and if no internal or external resorption is present, a root canal or standard endodontic procedure can typically be performed. Even routine endodontic procedures take specialized equipment and advanced skills, and complications can be common, so referral may be an option.

A basic description of the procedure (which you can use to inform your clients) includes: removal of the pulp (filing the canal); sterilization and irrigation; drying the canal; and placing a sealer cement and inert filling material (gutta percha) to fill and seal the region, particularly the apical region (Figure 5.2). The access and fracture sites are closed with a restorative (composite). The tooth is not vital but is still functional as long as the supporting periodontal structures are adequate. Metal crowns can be placed for additional protection, but many teeth can be maintained without them. Additional trauma (e.g., chewing hard objects) should be avoided.

Immature Teeth. If the pulp is nonvital but the apex is still open, an alternate procedure is needed to stimulate closure of the apex (*apexification*) before standard endodontics can be performed. A complete fill with calcium hydroxide paste to stimulate hard-tissue closure of the apex is placed every 6 months until the apex is solid enough for a complete seal. A nonvital deciduous tooth should be extracted.

ORTHODONTICS

Orthodontics is a very complicated field, but basic aspects can be evaluated here, and you can certainly take steps to alleviate discomfort or pain due to malocclusions. Although every patient may not need a perfect bite, each is certainly entitled to a comfortable and functional bite. Beyond that, there are ethical considerations concerning any procedure that would alter the appearance of a patient (standards of the American Veterinary Medical Association [AVMA], rules of the American Kennel Club [AKC], etc.). If any changes are made, an orthodontic release form stating that there is no intent of deceit should be signed by the owner.

Normal Occlusion

Many pets have occlusal variations that are relatively functional, but it is important to know what comprises a "normal occlusion" as a guideline for complete assessment (see Table 5.1).

Table 5.1
Orthodontic classification

Class	Description	Examples
0	Normal Breed normal	Normal Brachycephalic—boxer
I	Jaw relationship normal Individual tooth maloccluded	Base narrow Anterior crossbite Lance canine Posterior crossbite
II	Mandible short in relation to maxilla	Overbite Unilateral wry ($\frac{1}{2}$ mandible short)
III	Maxilla short in relation to mandible	Underbite Unilateral wry ($\frac{1}{2}$ maxilla short)
IV	Special malocclusion	Mixed wry ($\frac{1}{2}$ maxilla short with $\frac{1}{2}$ mandible long)

Incisor Relationship

In a proper jaw relationship, the incisors should fit in a *scissor bite,* with the upper incisor crowns *occluding* rostral to the lower incisors, without excessive gap. To limit your assessment to this aspect of occlusion, however, could be misleading.

Jaw Relationship

Most genetic occlusal variations deal with the relative length of the jaws. This can best be assessed by observing the premolar relationship. The upper and lower premolars should be spaced, for optimum shearing effect, with the tip of the cusp of a tooth in one arch pointing directly into the interdental space between two teeth of the opposite arch. This pinking-shear configuration provides optimum interdigitation. With the mouth slightly open, the *developmental grooves* of the carnassial teeth (upper fourth premolar and lower first molar) should line up, forming a diamond shape in the space (Figure 5.3).

Canine Relationship

Even with a normal scissor bite, the mandible can sometimes be slightly long (in comparison to the maxilla), so in addition to looking at the premolars, you can also evaluate the spacing of the canine teeth. The lower canine tooth should lie in the interdental *diastema* between the upper third incisor and canine, equidistant between the two teeth.

Carnassial Teeth Relationship

The great majority of dogs will have the upper fourth premolar crowns buccal to the lower first molars. Some breeds (e.g., collies) can have a *posterior crossbite,* with the lower molar crown situated buccally.

Figure 5.3 *Normal occlusion at carnassial teeth with developmental groove lining up*

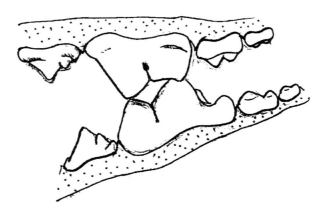

(Illustration adapted from original drawing by R. B. Wiggs)

Malocclusion

Any variation of the normal standards is considered a malocclusion. Some changes will not cause significant problems, but others require some form of intervention. Any advanced or complicated therapy should generally be performed by specialists. Orthodontic movement requires advanced knowledge and skill, specialized equipment, and an owner dedicated to frequent follow-up visits while anticipating potential complications.

Normal Jaw Relationship

When the jaw lengths are in correct proportion, there can still be influences—sometimes genetic but often developmental—that affect the position of individual teeth (Class I malocclusion). A common cause is the retention of deciduous teeth when the permanent teeth are erupting. If a deciduous tooth is still in place, the permanent tooth will be deflected into an abnormal position when it erupts (Figure 5.4).

Anterior Crossbite. This term refers to the condition in which one or more of the maxillary incisor teeth are positioned behind, or caudal to, the mandibular incisors (Figure 5.5). Incisors tend to be deflected lingually or palatally with persistent deciduous teeth, and once the interlock is physically in place, it is difficult for the tooth to move back on its own. This may predispose the individual to accelerated periodontal disease caused by crowding, improper occlusal forces, and inadequate use. Orthodontic movement using brackets and elastics or maxillary appliances to move the upper incisors further forward can be attempted.

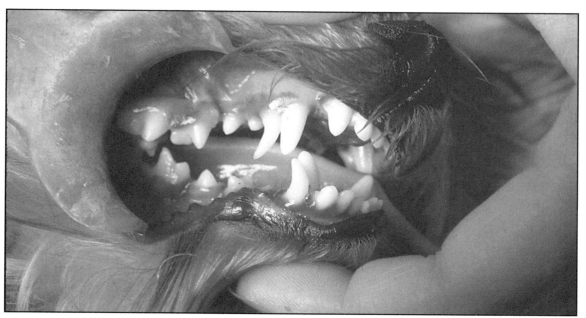

Figure 5.4 *Retained (persistent) deciduous teeth cause deflected eruption of permanent teeth*

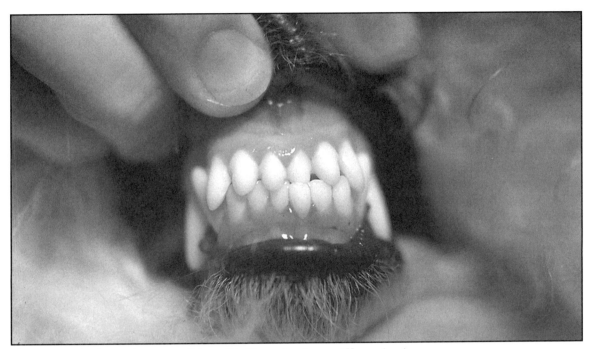

Figure 5.5 *Anterior crossbite of left central maxillary incisor*

Base Narrow Canines. Mandibular canines will be deflected lingually in the presence of retained deciduous teeth. This can position the teeth to erupt directly into the palate (Figure 5.6). If the tooth is barely catching the edge of the palatal gingiva, a *gingivectomy* to release the tooth may be sufficient (Figure 5.7). If the mandibular canine is traumatizing the palate, you can shorten the crown with amputation, and the pulp can be treated as if it were a recent canal exposure (see the preceding section on vital pulpotomy). Orthodontically, an *incline plane* can be fashioned either directly in the mouth with acrylics or composites or at an outside lab (metal appliance) (Figure 5.8). The goal is to redirect the angle of the tooth so it is "inclined" laterally into a more correct position. If unilateral, the incline plane might keep the bite open, preventing the opposite tooth from being secure in its diastema. Composite buildup on the crown can help hold it in place and keep the jaw from drifting to one side. This buildup can also be used on teeth that have not fully erupted to enhance their retention. One common problem occurs if the maxillary diastema between the upper third incisor and canine is too narrow for the lower canine to fit. Additional work would be needed in such a case.

Lance Teeth (Rostroversion). The maxillary canines will be deflected rostrally in the presence of persistent or retained deciduous teeth (Figure 5.9). If such eruption occurs early, the canine will block the diastema that is necessary for the placement of the lower canine. So, in addition to the maloccluded maxillary canine, the mandibular one can become *base narrow* or have a buccal

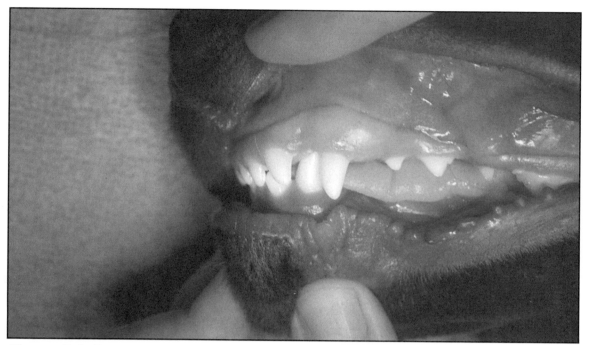

Figure 5.6 *Base narrow mandibular canine*

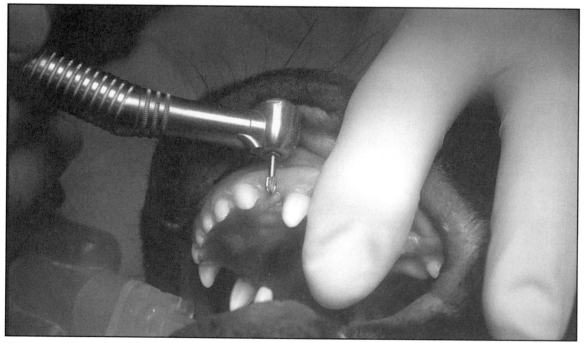

Figure 5.7a *Gingivectomy to release gingival impingement of base narrow canine*

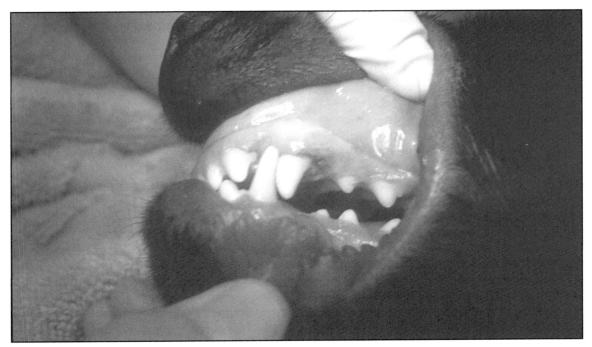

Figure 5.7b *Additional crown buildup with composite to help "retain" tooth*

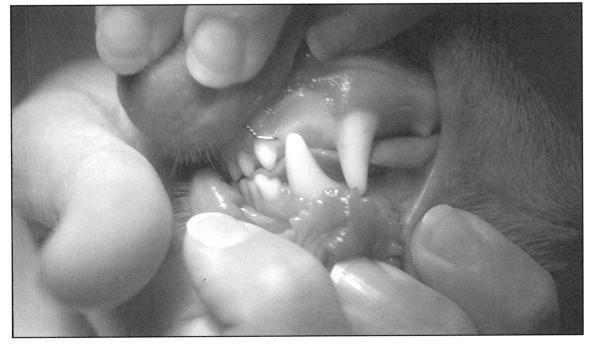

Figure 5.7c *Acrylic incline plane*

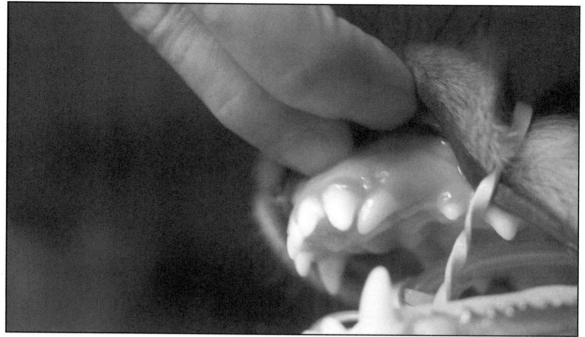

Figure 5.9 *Lance tooth (maxillary canine)*

deviation. Correction of the upper canine will often utilize orthodontic brackets or buttons on the upper fourth premolar and first molar as *anchorage* teeth, from which an elastic is stretched to a button on the maxillary canine, to apply force to move it backward. Some breeds (e.g., shelties) may have an exaggerated form of *lance tooth,* in which the canine erupts pointing directly forward, parallel to the ground.

 Posterior Crossbite. As described earlier, a posterior crossbite may just be an incidental finding, particularly in collies (Figure 5.10). Any form of orthodontic movement would be very complicated, as the mouth would have to be forced to remain open for a period of time to allow the teeth to "pass by" each other. You should instruct the owner to watch the area more closely for periodontal disease.

Abnormal Jaw Relationship
 With all of the different head shapes found in dogs and even cats, added to the fact that the four jaw quadrants are all genetically "coded" separately from each other, it is unusual to find a completely normal bite. Moreover, it would be impossible to try to return every individual to a normal occlusion, but do pay attention to any conditions that cause discomfort or compromise the health of the oral cavity, and take steps to lessen any significant problems.

 Breed "Normals" (Class 0 Malocclusion). Some degree of malocclusion is allowed as a breed standard for quite a few breeds. Such a condition should not be considered a true malocclusion, unless even the breed standard is

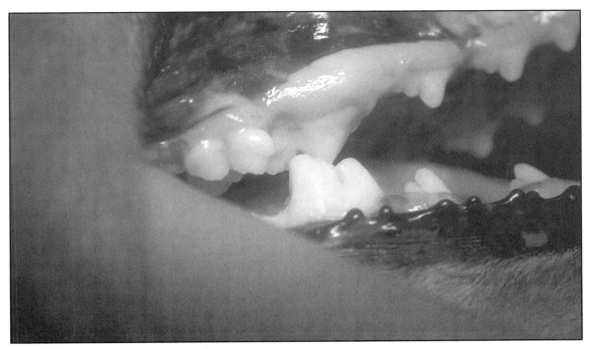

Figure 5.10 *Posterior crossbite*

exaggerated. It is interesting to note that many breed standards allow a *"level bite,"* in which the incisor tips meet each other, which can both be uncomfortable and cause excessive wear.

"Overbite" (Class II Malocclusion). In this classification, either the mandible is short in relation to the maxilla (mandibular brachygnathism—Figure 5.11) or the maxilla is too long (maxillary prognathism). The most significant problem arises when the lower canine is forced into a position level to or behind the upper canine, often causing it to hit the palate. Depending on the extent of the situation, the lower canine can be moved either rostrally and buccally or distally and buccally if closer to the distal aspect of the maxillary canine. Crown amputation and pulp capping may also be performed to resolve the traumatic occlusion. At times, the lower incisors will also hit the palate once the canine problem is corrected, so monitor them as well.

"Underbite" (Class III Malocclusion). Here, the mandible may be too long (mandibular prognathism), but often it is the maxilla that is too short (maxillary brachygnathism—*brachycephalic*), sometimes as a result of selective breeding. In mild cases, the only apparent sign may be a forward shift of the lower premolars with the lower canines hitting the upper corner incisors, and a scissor bite may be present (Figure 5.12). Often, the lower incisors are in front of the uppers, however, so trauma to the floor of the mouth and wear on the lingual aspect of the lower canines may occur. At times, the lower canine will hit the palate at the corner incisor, but extraction of the incisor will often provide sufficient space for the canine to move into (Figure 5.13).

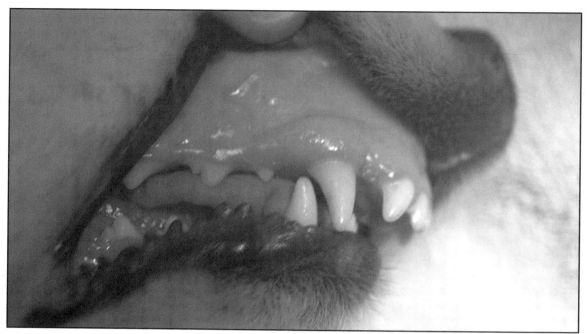

FFigure 5.11 *Class II malocclusion*

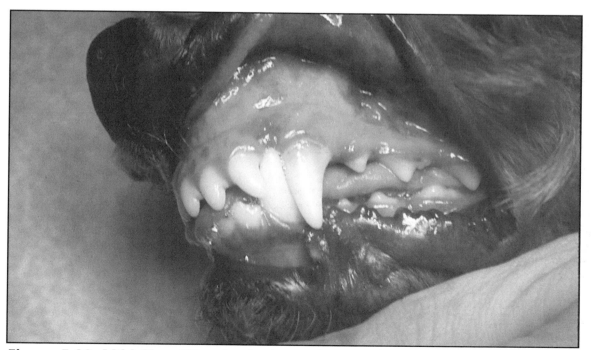

Figure 5.12 *Mild Class III malocclusion with the mandibular canine tight against maxillary corner incisor*

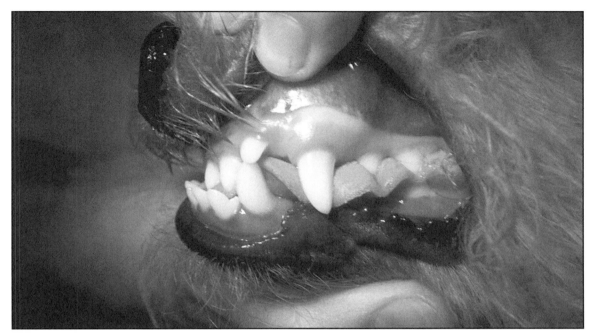

Figure 5.13a *Class III malocclusion with mandibular canines hitting corner incisors*

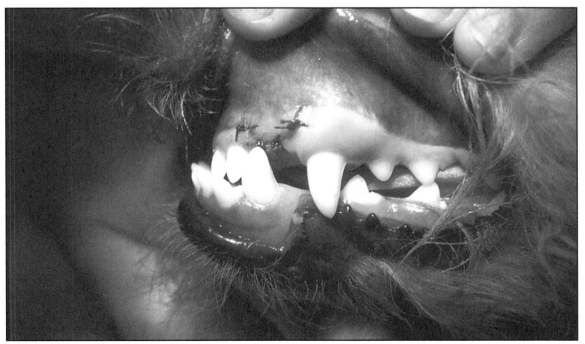

Figure 5.13b *Extraction of maxillary corner incisors to relieve occlusal trauma*

"Wry Bite" (Class IV Malocclusion). When one of the four jaw quadrants experiences abnormal growth (either excessive or insufficient), the midline of that arch will be altered (Figure 5.14). Lining up the symphyses (mandibular and maxillary) or the interdental space between the central incisors is one easy way to evaluate this condition. You may see an individual with one long quadrant and one short quadrant, which can contribute to a significant occlusal variation.

Immature Malocclusions

Deciduous teeth and jaws can experience many of the same malocclusions as seen in the adult oral cavity, but developmental changes and growth patterns can make management more interesting. Constant changes in the jaw-length relationship can occur, with mandibular growth typically finishing later. Orthodontic movement of deciduous teeth is rarely undertaken because the teeth will soon be exfoliated. Even with *exfoliation,* however, major problems can occur with deciduous malocclusions if abnormal interlocks of teeth against teeth or soft tissue interfere with normal jaw growth (Figure 5.15). If such an interlock should occur, extraction of the involved deciduous teeth would not necessarily cure the problem, but it would allow the jaws to grow into their genetic potential.

Anytime a mandibular deciduous canine is hitting the palate, whether in a simple *base narrow* condition or an advanced Class II malocclusion, extract it to relieve the impediment. Because of uncoordinated jaw growth spurts, the mandible is sometimes longer than the maxilla temporarily, even if the genetic potential is for a normal jaw relationship. If this causes the upper incisors to get "caught" behind the lower incisors, the

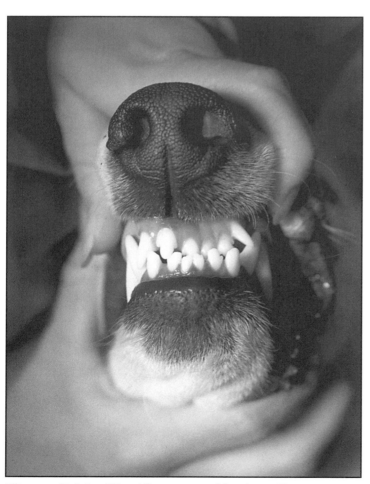

Figure 5.14a *Significant wry bite in a German shepherd dog*

general rule is to extract the incisors in the "shorter" jaw. The exception to this would be a condition in which the lower canine teeth are in contact with the upper corner incisors, in effect creating a beneficial interlock that could help keep the mandible from growing out even further! In other cases, a shortened mandible can cause the lower canines to occlude distal to the uppers. In such cases, you should extract the deciduous teeth to relieve the interlock (*interceptive orthodontics*) before permanent *tooth eruption* to allow for sufficient jaw growth and correction before the permanent teeth come into occlusion with each other (optimally at 8 to 11 weeks of age). Perform extractions *very* carefully (see chapter 4: Oral Surgery—

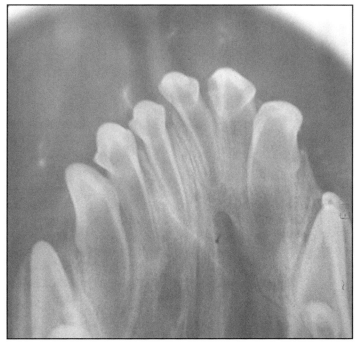

Figure 5.14b *Radiograph of wry bite, maxillary deviation*

Extraction), as any trauma can disturb the submerged permanent tooth bud and cause significant damage. Less than half of the dogs receiving interceptive orthodontics show improvement, but the others are genetically destined to have an abnormal occlusion anyway. In some cat breeds, such as Persians, it seems that temporary malocclusions often respond well to planned extractions, but again, it is the genetics behind the individual that determines final jaw growth.

RESTORATIVE DENTISTRY

Some aspects of restorative dentistry may deal with the aesthetic restoration of appearance, but most veterinary restorative attempts are intended to restore function and relieve discomfort. If the appearance is enhanced along the way and if there is no intent to hide an abnormality, then both the patient and the owner can be satisfied.

Resorptive Lesions

These lesions will be covered more extensively in regard to cats in chapter 7: Feline Oral and Dental Disease, but sometimes dogs can have similar lesions, primarily exhibited as internal resorption that may appear as a pinkish discoloration of the tooth (Plate 16). Radiographs, as always, are vital in

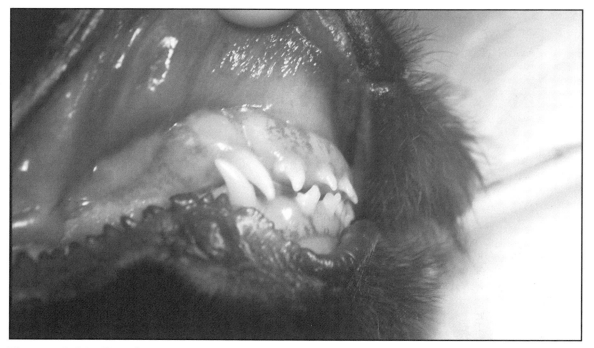

Figure 5.15 *Deciduous malocclusion with improper canine interlock; interceptive orthodontics (extraction) would be warranted*

making a complete assessment of the condition. With the larger teeth, if the root structure is healthy, endodontic therapy can remove the inflamed pulp, and the resorptive area may be restored with composites. Alternatively, the more severely affected portion of the tooth can be removed, preserving the remainder of the tooth with endodontics. If significant tooth structure is compromised and root resorption is present, simple restoration may not be an option. Extraction of these teeth can be even more challenging than in cats because ankylosis of the roots to the alveolar bone can anchor these teeth. With extensive involvement of multiple teeth, radical bone removal to extract all tooth substance can sometimes compromise the jaw. If significant root resorption with osseous remodeling is present without signs of periapical infection, remove as much tooth structure as possible without injuring the jaw, and pack an osseogenic substance before closure. If some root substance must be left, the records should indicate location, and the owner should be informed to ensure regular rechecks and radiographs. If there is any indication of periapical bone loss or soft-tissue inflammation, all tooth structure should be removed.

Carious Lesions (Cavities)

Because of many influences (amount of occlusal table, pH of saliva, amount of carbohydrates in diet), the incidence of caries in dogs is low, but occasional instances will be found. Typically, the occlusal surfaces of the molars are affected, possibly because food accumulates there. A higher incidence might be expected in animals who get softer diets or diets that contain higher amounts of refined carbohydrates (starches and sugars). The bacterial decay may start as a discolored section of enamel that is often softer than normal. The sharp point of an explorer will "stick" in this region. After a slow progression through the enamel, caries can extend quite rapidly through the softer dentin, forming a "mushroom" lesion and often exposing the pulp. Frequently, the carious lesion has extended into the tooth structure, and the chance of a simple restoration is diminished before being detected. If the lesion has not reached the pulp, cavity preparation to remove diseased tissue from the site precedes the application of a restorative, such as a composite. If the pulp is compromised but sufficient tooth structure is present, endodontic therapy is performed before restoration. Such techniques of restoration do require special materials and equipment.

Enamel Hypocalcification and Enamel Hypoplasia

As the permanent teeth are forming, many influences can affect the development of the tooth, especially the enamel. The condition is marked by pitting and discoloration of the teeth, sometimes because of systemic disease or fever (distemper teeth), and is more correctly termed *enamel hypocalcification*. This poorly mineralized enamel will wear and chip off the teeth more easily, causing a very rough surface. This effect may be magnified in dogs who are heavy chewers, especially "cage-biters" who wear down the distal aspects of their canine teeth (Figure 5.16). Treatment consists of enamel scrubbing—gently removing areas of diseased enamel while retaining as much normal tissue as possible. The most accurate instruments to use include white stone burs or finishing discs on a high-speed handpiece with water, but even sonic and ultrasonic scalers will remove some of the soft enamel and smooth the surfaces. Care should be used with the ultrasonic scaler, particularly with the temperature of the tip. If the condition is generalized, a good bonding agent may be applied to treat the potentially sensitive areas of exposed dentin. A strong, in-clinic fluoride may also help, and regular home care with brushing and weekly application of stannous fluoride (avoid excessive ingestion, or if inadequate kidney function) can reduce discomfort and minimize periodontal inflammation. Focal areas of enamel defects can be restored with flowable composites for increased aesthetics. All affected teeth should be radiographed because some roots may be affected as well, making the long-term prognosis poor. Regular teeth cleaning should be performed, with removal of enamel that has subsequently become involved.

Fractured Crown with No Canal Exposure

If small portions of a tooth crown are fractured without exposing the canal, attention should be paid to the lesion even if it doesn't seem to bother the pet. Actually, the exposed dentinal tubules can cause some sensitivity, and every damaged tooth should be radiographed to look for any hidden trauma.

Restorations on a vital tooth should entail more precautions, such as limiting the use of acid etching materials on the dentinal tubules and avoiding

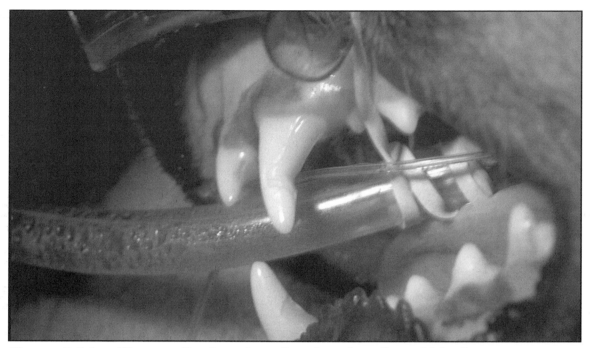

Figure 5.16a *Wear on distal surface of canines from "cage biting"*

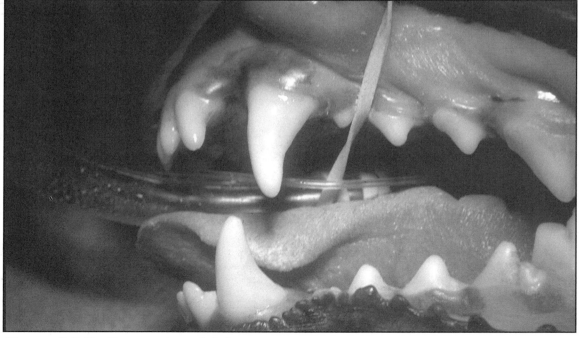

Figure 5.16b *Restoration of defect*

excessive heat generation with burs. The rough edges of the fracture site should be smoothed down (with a white stone bur), with a bevel finish given to the enamel edges. A bonding agent can be placed on its own over the fracture site or as the first step in a composite restorative. Sufficient composite should be placed on the tooth to restore its rounded, smooth contour, with smooth margins, even if it is shorter than the opposite tooth. Any material placed on the tooth should not go beyond the height of the remaining crown; if it is, it can easily be broken off, and future tooth trauma should be avoided whenever possible. Radiographs on subsequent follow-ups are also recommended, as the pulp could still be compromised from the trauma even if it wasn't exposed, and it could eventually die.

Prosthodontics

The area of prosthodontics is probably the most specialized in veterinary dentistry, requiring advanced skills and specific instrumentation, including the use of a dental laboratory to manufacture devices such as crowns, veneers, bridges, and implants.

Crowns

Although many of these items may be considered elective choices, crowns are placed for additional protection of teeth that need to remain functional in certain working dogs (Figure 5.17). Some dogs who are heavy chewers may also benefit from metal crowns placed on carnassial teeth if their behavior cannot be completely modified. Owners need to know that crowns are not indestructible. Crowns made of porcelain fused to metal and Inceram (Viadent, Brea, CA) crowns provide a more normal-looking tooth.

Implants and Bridges

When a tooth has been completely lost in human dentistry, it is commonly replaced with a bridge or implant, both to restore function and enhance the patient's self-esteem. Fortunately, given the difficulty of making such devices succeed, the aesthetic aspect in veterinary medicine is not as significant; indeed, the indications for such devices may be outweighed by the difficulty in making them successful. Implantology is an extremely specialized area, and the bone structure of dogs is not as amenable to this therapy as the human jaw. Bridges will typically be for used aesthetics only, as the forces in a canine mouth can prove damaging to any prosthetic device.

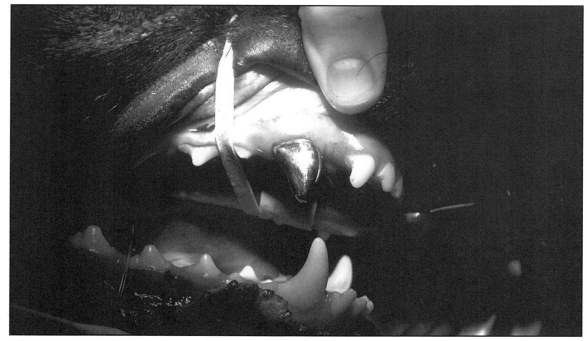

Figure 5.17   *Metal crown restoration on Belgian Malinois cuspid*

MAJOR ORAL SURGERY

Some aspects of routine oral surgery have been covered in a previous chapter (see chapter 4: Oral Surgery). More advanced procedures for tumor removal (the various "ectomies") can be found in the many surgery and dental texts that cover these topic in depth. Some surgical procedures are also covered in the emergency section of this volume (see chapter 6: Oral and Dental Emergencies).

Oral and Dental Emergencies

As a general rule, most oral and dental emergencies fall into one of several categories: infection, inflammation, resorption, or trauma. Dental emergencies among pets are seldom life-and-death matters, but they generally are conditions that need some form of immediate care to alleviate pain, stabilize an injury, or salvage oral structures. Many of the emergency treatments are only temporary in nature, designed to stabilize the patient or dental condition before instituting a more complete treatment program at a later time. However, in some cases, either because of convenience, speed, or necessity, full care must be given on the initial visit after the emergency occurs. Therefore, you must be able to quickly assess and separate emergencies from nonemergencies.

Emergency treatment of most of these conditions does not necessarily require a specialist or much in the way of special equipment. Although an oral examination may provide most of the information required, oral and dental X rays may be needed to fully diagnose the problem and develop a treatment plan (see chapter 2: Oral Examination and Recognition of Pathology—Radiology).

Infections that are considered emergencies may involve sudden cellulitis, abscess, pain, bleeding, or tooth loss. Inflammation and resorption may be found in either infection or trauma; in some cases, they are not necessarily found with either condition but in their own groupings. For simplicity, we will include them in the category of infection.

TRAUMA

Trauma is a common cause of oral and dental emergencies. The traumatic condition may encompass lacerations, degloving, burns, injured teeth, or fractures of the jaws.

Lacerations

Damage to the lips, oral mucosa, gums (gingiva), and tongue sometimes requires emergency wound treatment.

Treatment

One of your first tasks will be to control hemorrhage, while trying to not compromise normal blood flow to the tissues. The severity of the hemorrhage generally determines which treatment is required, from gentle pressure to the use of hemostasis solutions and even the ligation of vessels. This is part of the stabilization of the patient, which also includes monitoring vital signs and running emergency blood work and diagnostic tests such as radiographs and electroencephalographs (EKGs) to determine the extent of the injury and assess the patient's condition. You may need to start supportive care, such as intravenous fluids, plasma, or blood, or administer emergency medication. You can minimize immediate posttrauma swelling by applying cold packs (for minor cases), light pressure, or anti-inflammatory drugs. Pain management may include topical or local anesthetics to augment injectable analgesics for reduction of the patient's discomfort. In injuries that require more extensive work or with fractious animals, you may need to use some form of sedation or anesthesia, with appropriate indications.

Cleanse, disinfect, and debride the wound as needed. In traumatic wounds, you must always consider the injury contaminated, and every reasonable effort should be made to decontaminate it. Carefully remove any debris around vessels, nerves, or other vital structures. Necrotic tissue should also be removed judiciously. You can remove larger pieces of debris with tissue forceps and use warm saline lavage to irrigate the area to remove smaller debris. Wound closure is dependent upon the age, size, location, and extent of the wound. Primary closure is always desirable, but in some cases, delayed closure or secondary-intention healing may be best. On occasion, various flap closures or even free grafts may be required. Placement of drain tubes in contaminated wounds is not uncommon. The actual type of suture material used is generally based on the surgeon's preference. Home care and medications are dependent upon the patient, category of wound, and type of closure performed. Generally, antibiotics and pain management drugs will be part of the required home-care regimen.

The normal steps in treating lacerations follow:

- Control hemorrhage
- Stabilize patient
- Control swelling
- Implement pain management
- Clean and debride wound, removing necrotic tissue and debris and using antiseptic solutions and drain placement
- Close wound
- Instruct owner on home care

Degloving or Labial Avulsion of the Mandible

Degloving is typically associated with some form of trauma to the mandible that results in the labial skin of the lower jaw being stripped back under itself. It is not uncommon for additional oral injuries, such as broken teeth or jaw fractures, to be present, all of which must be addressed.

Treatment

The basic treatment is the same as that for soft-tissue lacerations, as previously described. Thoroughly cleanse and debride the wound. Next, reattach the subcutaneous tissues along the midline facia of the mandibular symphysis with absorbable suture material. Then, reposition the lip with a mattress suture pattern. In some cases, the tension on the lip can be considerable, and additional suture support may be required. In such a case, make a horizontal suture pattern into the subcutaneous tissues of the lower lip, with the wires or sutures brought up and around the canine teeth for a stronger anchorage.

The normal steps in treating degloving or labial avulsion injuries follow:

- Control hemorrhage
- Stabilize patient
- Control swelling
- Implement pain management
- Cleanse and debride wound
- Reattach subcutaneous tissues
- Reattach lip

Foreign Bodies

Some more inquisitive patients can end up with all kinds of foreign objects in the oral cavity—caught in the lips, the tongue, and even the palate.

Treatment

Carefully remove the foreign body, with minimal damage to surrounding structures. Evaluate the affected tissues, debriding any necrotic tissue or debris and flushing with antiseptic solutions where indicated. If similar objects can be encountered by the pet again, instruct the owner to keep them out of the pet's reach.

The normal steps in treating injuries caused by foreign bodies follow:

- Remove foreign body
- Treat affected tissues

Wounds

Wounds, abrasions, or ulcerations are generally traumatic in nature, but they can also occur because of exposure to chemicals or other irritants. Open epithelial injuries may require therapy.

Treatment

Mild abrasions or wounds can be treated conservatively by cleaning the wound and applying 3 to 6 layers of tincture of myrrh and benzoin as a gingival dressing. In more severe wounds, the area should be cleansed and sutured if possible. Instruct the owner on management at home with oral hygiene solutions, medications for pain management, and antibiotics when indicated. Maintaining oral comfort will be important to avoid anorexia.

The normal steps in treating wounds follow:

- Clean wound and dress
- Suture if necessary
- Instruct owner on home management

Burns

Oral electrical burns may be found on any mucosal surface and can vary in severity. Most 220- to 280-V insults are fatal to the pet, but 110- to 140-V injuries can result in treatable lesions.

Treatment

Observe the patient closely for secondary complications of pulmonary edema or cranial swelling, and treat these conditions accordingly should they arise. The actual burns should be treated conservatively for several weeks until their full extent can be determined. The radius of tissue injury from electrical insult can initially be obscure and difficult to evaluate. Surgical debridement and flaps may be required at some point, staged according to the defect encountered. Provide adequate pain management and home support, including nutritional supplementation if eating is difficult.

The normal steps in treating burns follow:

- Stabilize patient
- Manage burn—complete staged debridement
- Provide owner with information on home care and pain management

Palatal Trauma

Some palatal defects may be caused by oronasal fistulation resulting from periodontal disease or complications from extractions, but trauma can certainly compromise the integrity of the palate. Midline defects from automobile accidents or falls are palatal defects that warrant emergency treatment.

Treatment

Traumatic palatal injuries, when treated immediately, respond well to simple flap closures and suturing. Simple apposition with sutures may be adequate, or you may have to raise a flap for more complete closure (Figure 6.1).

The normal steps in treating palatal trauma follow:

- Suture midline defect close
- Assess for any additional injury

Injuries to Teeth

Teeth can encounter all kinds of trauma, be it from external sources or from chewing on hard objects. The extent of injury depends on the insult and the tooth's reaction to it.

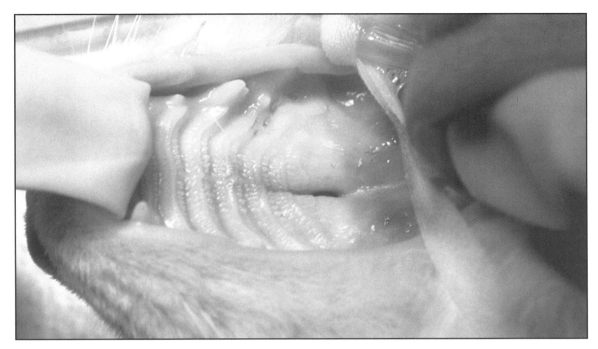

Figure 6.1a *Palatal defect, midline*

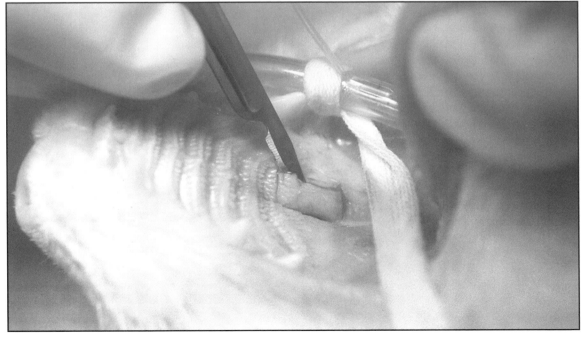

Figure 6.1b *Palatal flap for repair*

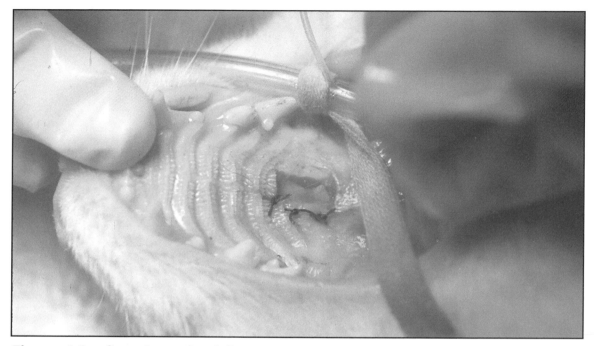

Figure 6.1c *Suturing palatal flap*

Discolored Teeth (Pulpitis)

Rose-, blue-, and beige-colored teeth are manifestations of different stages or phases of the same problem—internal tooth injury. Some form of injury to the tooth results in internal tooth hemorrhage within the pulp cavity. Sudden movements of the tooth that disrupt or sever the vessels entering the apex of the tooth to feed the pulp are the most common cause. The visible discoloration indicates the death of odontoblasts within the dentin and probably of the pulp within the pulp cavity. Initially, the tooth will be pink- or rose-colored (pulpitis), but with time and deterioration of the blood cells and pigments trapped within the tooth, it will begin to turn blue and finally assume a beige to rust-brown color. Some teeth with mild injuries may have a *reversible pulpitis,* and antibiotics and anti-inflammatory drugs may be beneficial in these cases. The darker discoloration usually indicates that these teeth are nonvital or dying internally. Evaluation with radiographs can help you determine tooth status.

The normal steps in treating injuries to the teeth follow:

- *Reversible pulpitis*: Medicate and then evaluate at a later date
- *Irreversible pulpitis*: Extract or perform endodontics (see chapter 5: Advanced Oral and Dental Problems—Endodontics)

Fractures of the Tooth Crown

These fractures are often discovered incidentally on physical exam or during routine therapy, but some individuals with crown fractures will show significant discomfort and require immediate attention. Fractures are typically staged according to the degree of injury to help determine the best course of treatment. The treatments that follow are geared to permanent teeth, as most seriously fractured deciduous teeth are typically best extracted.

Stage I. In stage I fractures, usually only a chip of enamel is broken off the tooth, and the tooth is still vital, but the edge can be rough and irritating. Smooth the rough enamel edges, and seal exposed dentinal tubules with a heavy fluoride treatment or application of several layers of a *dentinal bonding agent*.

Stage II. This type of fracture will remove a section of enamel and a portion of the dentin without exposing the pulp chamber, retaining the pulp vitality. Smooth and seal the fracture site, and consider applying a restorative material, such as composite.

Stage III. When a fracture of the tooth removes both enamel and dentin, exposing the root canal, and the pulp is still vital, you need to determine the proper therapy. In young animals or for a recent exposure, keeping the pulp vital may be beneficial (see chapter 5: Advanced Oral and Dental Problems—Vital Pulpotomy). The prognosis of this procedure decreases in older animals, and if keeping the pulp vital is not selected, either standard endodontics or extraction would be the next choice.

Stage IV. With canal exposure caused by a fracture through the enamel and the dentin or with a nonvital tooth whose pulp is dead or dying (and, in fact, even with an intact nonvital tooth), the therapy choices are limited to standard endodontics or extraction. With immature, nonvital teeth, apexification may be necessary (see chapter 5: Advanced Oral and Dental Problems—Endodontics).

Fractures of the Root

These fractures are staged for treatment by several factors: the tooth, the type of tooth, the location of the fracture, and the stability of the crown. The treatments that follow are again aimed primarily at permanent teeth, as deciduous teeth are typically best extracted when injured to any degree.

Root Fracture near the Gingival Sulcus When Crown Is Unstable. With any amount of instability, extraction is the treatment of choice (see chapter 4: Oral Surgery—Extractions).

Root Fracture in Midroot Area When Crown Is Stable. The alveolar bone will act as a splint for the root while odontoblasts make reparative dentin, so no therapy may be necessary. If there is any instability, you can apply a splint to attach the crown to adjacent teeth for 4 to 6 weeks to allow healing. Once the segment is stable, you can remove the splint. Extraction is always an option to resolve the problem.

Luxations

Luxations are typically caused by trauma, but some teeth may be predisposed to luxation by periodontal disease. In this condition, the teeth have been moved from their proper position in the alveolus but are still attached. If the luxation is a result of advanced periodontal disease, extraction is the only option, but if there are no complicating factors, you can attempt to retain the tooth. A tooth may also be invulsed with force and should be treated appropriately.

Treatment. It is important to clean the tooth socket of all debris, being sure to irrigate with sterile saline. You should also gently clean the tooth root and flush it with dexamethasone, but *do not* remove any periodontal ligament fragments. Replace the tooth within the socket, and reestablish the animal's normal occlusion. Some teeth can be stabilized simply by suturing the tears in the oral mucosa associated with the luxation. However, wiring (using a figure eight between the canine teeth or an Ivy Loop with other teeth) or use of an acrylic or temporary composite splint may be required (Figure 6.2). Splints should be left in place until the tooth becomes stable, usually for 3 to 6 weeks. Antibiotics and anti-inflammatory drugs can help reduce infection and inflammation. Because the blood supply to the tooth was disrupted, a standard endodontic procedure (root canal) needs to be done 2 weeks after the initial injury to avoid periapical infection (see chapter 5: Advanced Oral and Dental Problems—Endodontics).

The normal steps in treating a luxation follow:

- Clean the socket of all debris and flush with saline
- Clean the root and flush with dexamethasone
- *Do not* remove the periodontal ligament fragments
- Replace and stabilize tooth (for 3 to 6 weeks)

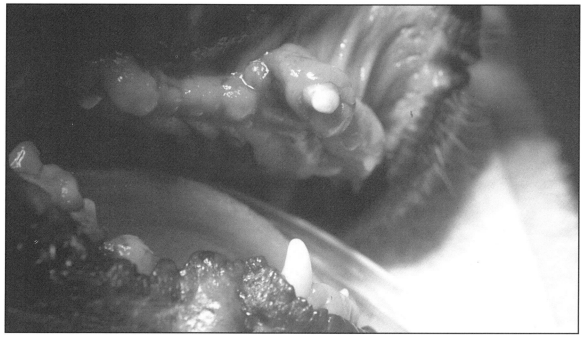

Figure 6.2a *Luxation or partial avulsion of right maxillary canine*

- Administer or prescribe antibiotics and anti-inflammatory drugs
- Perform standard endodontics within 2 weeks

Complete Tooth Avulsion

When a tooth is completely avulsed (not just luxated), or totally removed from the alveolar socket, the damage can be more significant. Most tooth avulsions are traumatic in origin, although certain conditions that weaken the alveolar bone, such as periodontal disease, can predispose a pet to this condition. Teeth avulsed due to periodontal disease should not be replanted, and you should treat the alveolus by cleaning it well and packing an osseogenic material before closure. This therapy may also be the choice with a simple traumatic avulsion if advanced therapy is not selected.

Tooth Reimplantation Treatment. One of the most important factors in the success of treating avulsed teeth is the proper and timely handling of the tooth. Reimplant the tooth as soon as possible. The longer the tooth is out of the mouth and the dryer it becomes, the less chance there is for reimplantation to succeed over the long term. Have the owners keep the tooth moist until brought to the clinic for reimplantation. Should the periodontal ligament (PDL) dry out, the success rate drops. The owners can place the tooth in fresh cold milk or cold water or simply wrap it in plastic wrap or aluminum foil to prevent rapid drying of the tooth. At the clinic, keep the tooth wrapped in gauze soaked in a sterile saline solution. Once you have the patient and tooth with you, therapy will be similar to that for a luxated tooth (see preceding section).

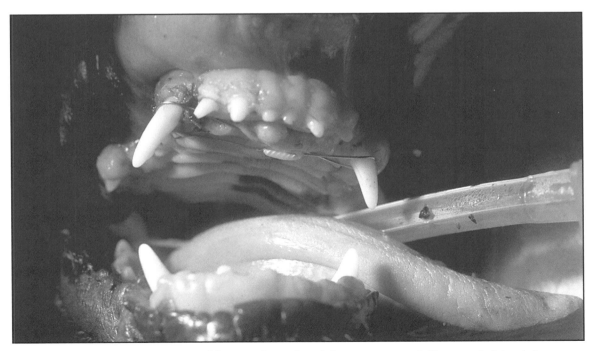

Figure 6.2b *Replacement of luxated tooth with sutures and figure-eight wiring*

The normal steps in treating a complete tooth avulsion follow:

- Clean the socket of all debris and flush with saline
- Clean the root and flush with dexamethasone
- *Do not* remove the periodontal ligament fragments
- Replace and stabilize tooth (for 3 to 6 weeks)
- Administer or prescribe antibiotics and anti-inflammatory drugs
- Perform standard endodontics within 2 weeks

Injuries Caused by Teeth (Malocclusions)

These conditions are seldom of a true emergency nature, except in the mind of distraught owners who have overlooked the condition until some sign or symptom alerts them to the problem. Many malocclusions of the teeth can result in self-trauma to the pet, and the most common ones are described in the orthodontics section (see chapter 5: Advanced Oral and Dental Problems—Orthodontics, especially the sections on lance tooth and base narrow mandibular canines). If a traumatized tooth causes an abnormal occlusion, you should attempt to correct it immediately.

Subluxated Tooth Malocclusion

This type of malocclusion typically occurs when a root is partially luxated from the alveolus because of trauma or advanced periodontal disease. The subluxated tooth then can block normal occlusion. Fractures of the alveolus, tooth crown, or tooth root are not uncommon in these conditions. To remove the trauma, you can either reimplant the tooth or extract it.

Jaw Fractures

Whenever there is facial or oral injury, you should evaluate all osseous structures for any fractures or injury. One of the most important things to remember about fracture repair is to maintain proper occlusion with reduction and stabilization.

Maxillary Fractures

Fractures of the upper jaw are most commonly caused by some form of trauma. There are many thin bones in the maxillary area that can be easily injured, and the degree of injury can vary greatly. Soft-tissue palate injuries, tooth luxations, oronasal communications, nasal passage obstruction, malocclusion, and facial disfigurement may occur, though the injuries are usually not complicated.

Treatment. With most maxillary fractures, you can provide stabilization with an acrylic splint or *osseous wiring* techniques (see treatment that follows). Extract or replace any teeth that are causing obstruction or interfering with normal occlusion. Suture any soft-tissue injuries, including any oronasal communication. Nasal obstructions may require surgical intervention if they cannot be reduced with the use of a blunt nasal probe.

The normal steps in treating maxillary fractures follow:

• Reduce and stabilize fracture
• Extract or replace teeth
• Suture soft tissue, including oronasal defects

Mandibular Fractures

Fractures of the mandible are also most commonly the result of some form of injury, though other factors can predispose an area to pathological fracture. Fractures of this nature are generally the result of some degree of alveolar bone loss caused by periodontal disease, tooth loss or extraction sites, or some generalized disease effecting mineralization (nutritional, endocrine). The weakened bone is vulnerable to stress that may occur with fighting or play (tug-of-war) that uses the teeth, simple mastication, or tooth extraction. In extractions, even delicate manipulation can result in a fracture if the bone has been seriously compromised, and forceful extraction techniques can easily fracture the bones of almost any jaw. In most cases, teeth involved in a fracture site should be retained, at least temporarily, to assist in the stabilization of the region (via wiring, use of splints). Once the fracture site is healed, select extraction or endodontics may be performed on teeth that have compromised pulps.

Symphysis Fracture or Separation. The symphysis area is the most frequently fractured region in cats, but it is a less common location in dog injuries (Figure 6.3). For treatment, reduce the fracture, and try to achieve as normal an occlusion as possible. In dogs with intact incisors, you may try a wire technique or an acrylic or temporary composite splint. In cats or if incisors are not stable, a circumferential wire technique placed behind the canines can reduce the fracture adequately. A strong suture material or wire in a modified figure-eight suture pattern can also be helpful. Don't tighten the wire excessively, as that will cause the lower canines to come in too far medially.

Fractures of the Body of the Mandible (Horizontal Ramus). Fractures in this area have a tendency to be categorized according to location and direction of the fracture. Anterior fractures are typically considered to be those in front of the third premolar, and posterior fractures are those behind it. A *favorable fracture* is one that helps hold the jaw segments together as the muscles of the lower jaw open the jaw, and an *unfavorable fracture* is one that is drawn apart by this action. A favorable fracture line is one that runs from the top of the mandible to the bottom in an anterior direction. An unfavorable fracture line is one that runs from the top of the mandible to the bottom in a posterior direction.

Reduce the fracture, and try to achieve as normal an occlusion as is possible. If most of the teeth are intact, a wiring technique (Stout's Multiple Loop) or a splint can be used to stabilize the fracture. If there are few teeth present, osseous, transosseous, or circumferential wiring techniques may be necessary to achieve stability. In comminuted fractures, a tape muzzle can be used to minimize mobility of the jaw if complete stability cannot be attained, or a

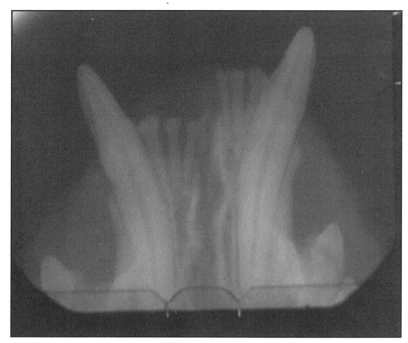

Figure 6.3a *Radiograph of mandibular symphysis fracture in a cat*

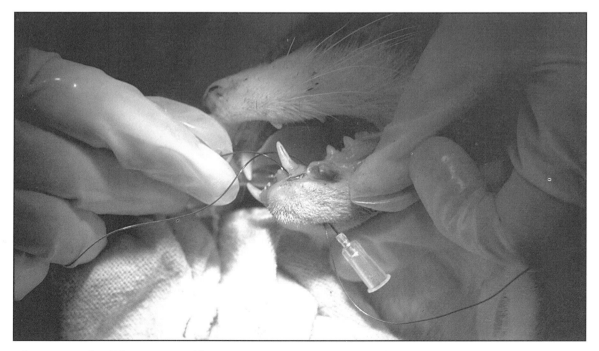

Figure 6.3b *Placement of large-gauge suture material*

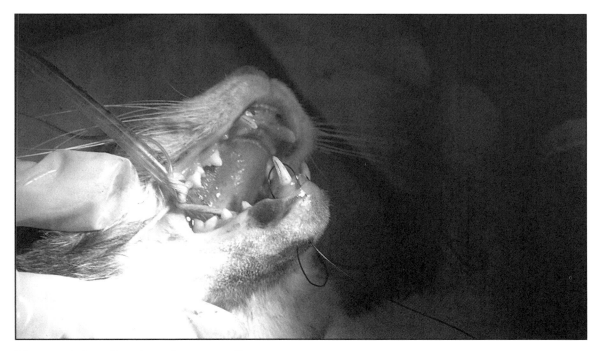

Figure 6.3c *Continued suture placement*

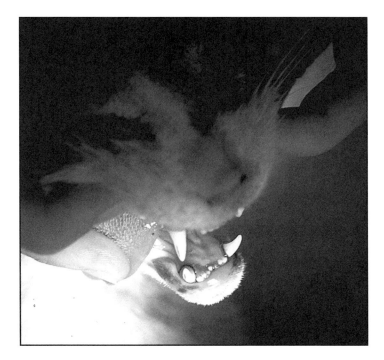

Figure 6.3d *Stabilization with suture tied in buried figure-eight pattern*

tape muzzle can be used in minor, nondisplaced fractures or even as an ancillary support for other methods.

Fractures of the Vertical Ramus, Condyloid Process, and Temporomandibular Joint. Injuries of the vertical ramus are usually of a traumatic nature, and other complicating injuries may be present and require additional emergency attention. These regions may be difficult to reach surgically, and if the fracture is minor or not displaced, you may select a more conservative treatment (e.g., a tape muzzle) to keep the area relatively stable.

Treatment

The many methods of treating fractures in the oral cavity can be found in surgical and dental texts. An important point in reduction and stabilization is to retain proper occlusion and function of the oral cavity. The endotracheal tube can be placed through a pharyngotomy incision to facilitate oral access and occlusal reconstruction. Often, however, more conservation methods of reduction can be very effective, if sufficient patient support, including adequate nutritional intake, is provided. In fact, many of the more invasive techniques of fracture stabilization (pins, plates, screws, etc.) can cause extensive damage to oral structures such as roots, vessels, and nerves (Figure 6.4).

Wiring Techniques. Most wiring methods are technique-sensitive and require additional experience and training (see the References and Recommended Readings section at the end of the book). Interdental wiring

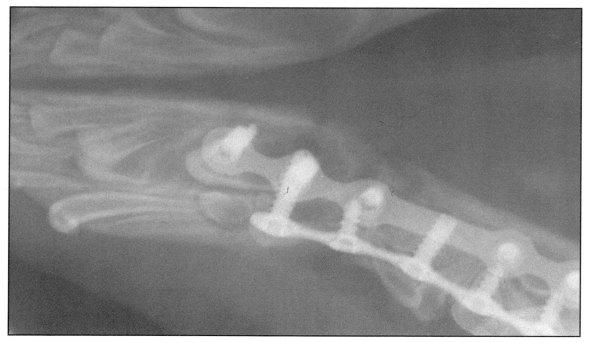

Figure 6.4 *Plate stabilization in a young dog's mandibular fracture has damaged permanent tooth buds*

techniques such as the Stout's Multiple Loop can provide excellent stability without rigidity and are minimally invasive. Osseous wiring techniques are often necessary when there are not sufficient teeth present for wiring or splinting, and they definitely require radiography for the correct placement of wires. Circumferential wiring is often helpful in symphyseal fractures, and they can be supplemented by a figure-eight pattern around the lower canines or incorporated into splints.

Splints. Acrylic or composite splints can be formed directly in the oral cavity to stabilize the reduced fracture, and incorporating wires around teeth and into the material can enhance retention of the splint. When using acrylics, be sure to protect the surrounding soft tissue with petroleum jelly, and use small amounts of powder and then liquid in a "salt and pepper" technique to avoid excessive heat production. Excessive use of dentinal bonding agents with composites can make splint removal more difficult and cause tooth staining, so use them in moderation (use caution with fumes).

The normal steps in treating mandibular fractures with splints follow:

- Reduce fracture, maintaining occlusion
- Place acrylic or composite incorporating teeth on either side of fracture
- Reinforce with wires

Interarch Stabilization. For comminuted fractures or those that are not easily splinted, stability of the jaws can be obtained by immobilizing the mouth with materials that secure the canine teeth to each other, allowing enough space so that the pet can lap up water and food. You can place a composite "bridge" between the upper and lower canines on both sides, leaving enough room for the patient to lap up water and a liquefied diet. The dental arches can also be stabilized with osseous wiring.

Tape Muzzle. As mentioned previously, you can provide conservative restriction of oral activity with a tape muzzle in comminuted fractures or as ancillary support for other means of stabilization. Pets with medium to long hair may need to be clipped to ease application and improve hygiene during the time of healing. Determine an oral opening with proper occlusion at the anterior teeth that would allow the animal to use its tongue to lap water and softened diets. According to the size of the pet, this will typically be between ¼ in. to ¾ in. Use a roll of 1-in. waterproof tape for constructing the tape muzzle. No tape will be directly stuck to the animal in this technique, although with difficult patients the tape may be reversed to stick to the pet for additional security.

The principal location for placement of the section around the muzzle is immediately behind the canine or cuspid teeth. Measure the distance from that point around the back of the head below the ears to the same location on the opposite side of the head. Cut a neck strap section of the tape two and a half times this length, and set it aside for later use. Wrap the tape around the muzzle, sticky side out, two times around, leaving sufficient laxity to allow the mouth to open slightly. Take the neck strap section of the tape, and with the sticky side out, center it behind the ears and bring it forward on both sides to the muzzle section. Apply a section of tape over the muzzle section of tape, this time with the sticky side in, entrapping the neck strap tape with two laps of the tape, and cut the roll of tape free. Next, fold the neck strap tape back over the muzzle strap and upon itself, so that the two sticky sides of the neck strap make contact. There should be a slight overlap of the two ends in the back. With no adhesive sides exposed, this allows the muzzle to be removed when required for examination or cleaning. Pain management procedures should be instituted. Some animals may also require sedation or tranquilization for a few days until they become accustomed to the oral restraint.

The normal steps in making a tape muzzle follow:

- Initially wrap muzzle to allow some oral opening
- Have the neck strap preplaced (from neck to muzzle wrap)
- Again wrap muzzle to secure neck strap
- Double back on neck strap

Salvage Procedures. When the bone has been badly damaged in the area, without a chance at stabilization, removing portions of the mandible can provide a functional oral cavity. This is sometimes accompanied by cheiloplasty to reduce the size of the oral orifice in the corners of the mouth in order to help support the jaw in a more natural alignment.

Temporomandibular Joint Dysfunction

Traumatic injuries to the distal portion of the mandible can cause injury to any portion of the temporomandibular joint (TMJ), from fracture to luxation. Individual laxity of the joints or even degenerative changes can cause problems as well.

Locking-Jaw Syndromes

Any interference with the normal function of the TMJ can result in occlusal interference or even locking of the jaw (open-mouth jaw locking). Take radiographs to establish the exact syndrome or injury present. A partial differential diagnosis would be flaring of the coronoid process, partially luxated or displaced tooth malocclusion, fracture of jaw, dislocation of the TMJ, and malocclusion. Each is addressed within this chapter.

Fractures of the Condyloid Process or TMJ. If there is minimal displacement and the fracture is stable, conservative treatment with a tape muzzle may provide the required stabilization. Unstable fractures that interfere with joint function are difficult to reduce and stabilize, so condylectomy may be required to restore some function. Even minor fractures that eventually heal may form a bony callous or experience degeneration that can diminish the range of motion.

The normal steps in treating fractures of the condyloid process or TMJ follow:

- Provide conservative support with minor fractures
- Perform a condylectomy if injury is severe or if it interferes with function

Luxation of the TMJ Joint. Sub- or total luxation of the TMJ is often the result of trauma, and the direction of the luxation may be ventral or rostral. For reduction of the luxation, you can use a wooden or plastic dowel pin approximately ¼ in. to ½ in. in diameter. Place the dowel pin between the developmental grooves of the upper and lower carnassial teeth (Figure 6.5). Then, gently press the rostral segments of the maxilla and mandible. If the TMJ luxation is reduced and the jaw is made functional once again, place a tape muzzle to maintain stability for 3 weeks, and initiate anti-inflammatories. If the luxation is not reduced or occurs again, the procedure can be repeated, but if additional attempts are unfruitful or any crepitation is felt, additional evaluation is needed. Chronic recurrences might indicate degenerative changes in the joint and might require condylectomy.

Figure 6.5 *Dowel placement for TMJ luxation reduction*

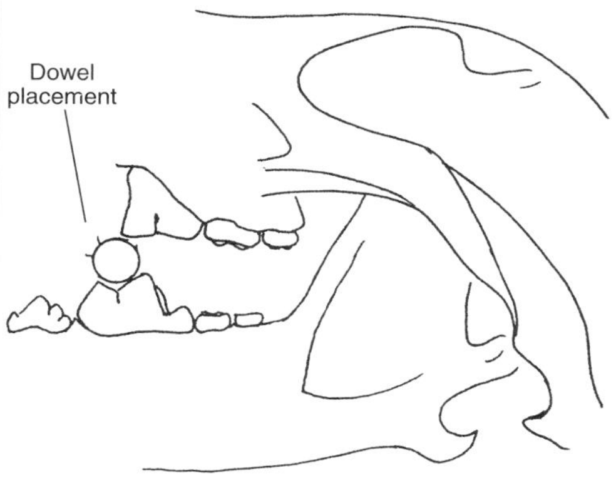

Dowel placement

(Illustration adapted from original drawing by R. B. Wiggs)

The normal steps in treating a luxation of the TMJ follow:

- Confirm luxation by radiography
- Place wooden dowel
- Reduce luxation with gentle pressure on anterior maxilla or mandible

Flaring of the Coronoid Process. This condition may mimic a luxation with the open-mouth locking, but simple dowel placement and reduction will not be effective treatments. In patients with this condition, there is probably an underlying laxity in the TMJ that allows some degree of lateral movement. With extreme mouth opening (yawning, meowing), there can be enough movement to allow the coronoid process to slip underneath the zygomatic arch and get "locked" out to it laterally. This can often be detected either by the obvious bulging of the cheek in the area of the zygomatic arch where the coronoid process is caught or by radiography (Figure 6.6).

Place gentle pressure on the coronoid process to guide it under the zygomatic arch, while opening the mouth further to allow the coronoid process to slip back

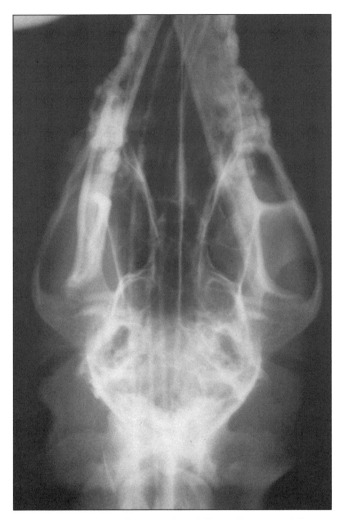

Figure 6.6 *Radiograph of flared coronoid process*

into place and permit the mouth to close properly. For a short period, use of a tape muzzle and anti-inflammatories will reduce the chance of recurrence, but because these conditions have a tendency to recur on a regular basis, surgical intervention may be necessary. It might be difficult to correct the underlying TMJ problem, so the effort is made to decrease the chance that locking will occur. You can do this by removing the ventral border of the zygomatic arch and, in some cases, even the dorsal border of the coronoid process (Figure 6.7). With the jaw in the locked position (and surgically prepped), you should remove part of the coronoid process first, before it slips back into place behind the zygomatic arch, at which time you can then work on the ventral zygomatic arch.

The normal steps in treating a flaring of the coronoid process follow:

- Confirm coronoid flare with palpation
- Conservatively reduce with lateral pressure on the flare while opening the mouth further
- Surgically correct with removal of ventral portion of zygomatic arch and dorsal border of coronoid process

Infections, Inflammations, and Resorptions

Although most conditions involving infections, inflammation, and resorption are not critical in nature, patients sometimes experience acute exacerbations of these conditions, requiring immediate relief. Once the emergency situation has been handled, follow-up therapy to deal with the complete treatment is recommended.

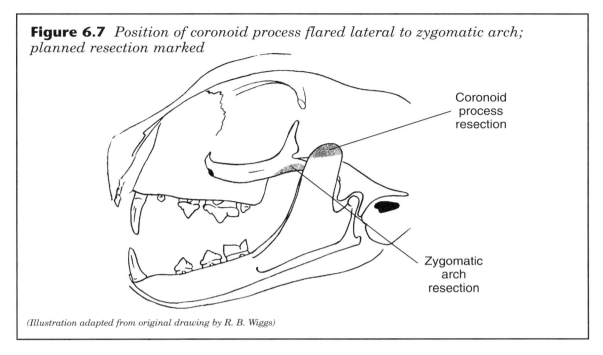

Figure 6.7 *Position of coronoid process flared lateral to zygomatic arch; planned resection marked*

Coronoid process resection

Zygomatic arch resection

(Illustration adapted from original drawing by R. B. Wiggs)

Endodontic Infections

Endodontic infections stem from bacterial assault on the pulp or the junction between the pulp and the periodontal tissues at the apex of the tooth. These endodontic infections may result in cellulitis, abscess with or without a draining tract, facial pain, lethargy, anorexia, and fever. Many endodontic infections are nearly subclinical, but when the signs appear acutely (Phoenix abscess), the condition can be quite painful. If an abscess is present, sedate the patient before lancing the lesion to allow drainage to relieve the pressure and begin a course of antibiotics and pain management. Final treatment (endodontics or extraction) may be decided on once the inflammation subsides.

The normal steps in treating an endontic infection follow:

• Assess patient and lance abscess
• Treat with antibiotics, and manage pain
• Schedule endodontics or extraction

Periodontic Infection

Periodontal infections generally result in periodontal abscesses, loss of tooth attachment, tooth mobility, deep periodontal pockets, tooth loss, oronasal fistula either with or without the tooth present, and, in some cases, bleeding from the mouth or nose. Again, though most problems are not emergencies, occasionally an abscessation can make a pet uncomfortable. The draining tract of a periodontal abscess can usually be differentiated on radiograph, but a general rule with permanent dentition is that most periodontal abscesses will be found and have their draining tracts at the mucogingival line or in the attached gingiva, whereas endodontic abscesses and their draining tracts are more commonly found above the mucogingival line on the alveolar mucosa (or their draining tracts will be somewhere on the face). Periodontal abscess are more commonly the result of calculus or foreign material being forced up into the gingiva or the periodontal ligament, thereby permitting bacteria to enter these tissues and result in infection and possibly an abscess. If focal in nature, the abscess can be lanced (at the site or through the gingival sulcus), and the lesion can be treated to salvage the tooth. Oral antibiotics as well as antibiotics packed into the sulcus may help reduce the bacterial infection. Once the inflammation has subsided, a complete periodontal assessment will help determine the most appropriate therapy. (see chapter 3: Periodontal Disease).

The normal steps in treating a periodontic infection follow:

- Assess abscess and lance if necessary
- Treat with site and oral antibiotics
- Institute periodontal therapy, if indicated, once inflammation subsides

Tooth Loss

If a tooth has been luxated or avulsed traumatically but was compromised due to periodontal disease, you shouldn't attempt to reimplant it. Clean the alveolus, and flush out any debris. If heavily infected, leave it open for drainage, but closure with osseogenic products and suturing a flap closed will provide a stronger alveolar ridge, if these procedures are possible. Use appropriate antibiotic therapy.

Oral or Nasal Bleeding

Bleeding can sometimes occur during advanced periodontal disease involving the maxillary canine teeth. As the periodontal disease approaches the tooth apex, it may cause the erosion of the support vessels near the tooth's apex. These vessels may suddenly rupture, resulting in bleeding either from the nose or the oral cavity. The condition must be differentiated from certain systemic infections, as well as infection or tumors of the nasal passage. Typically, if the condition is periodontal in nature, a periodontal probe can be inserted into a deep pocket on the palatal surface of the maxillary canine tooth and will probably enter the nasal passage through this pocket. In cases of this nature, the bleeding is normally of a relatively short to moderate duration, lasting from 1 to 8 hours typically. However, the amount of blood loss can sometimes appear to be substantial, causing serious owner concern, although no animal mortalities from this condition have been observed.

If there is bleeding from the nasal passage, the use of ice packs and nasal decongestant sprays into the affected nostril may reduce or control the bleeding. Once the patient is stabilized, you can extract the tooth, pack off the tooth socket with a product that aids in bone growth and healing (if it will be retained), and close the site with a gingival flap. Postoperative care will include antibiotics and pain management as required.

The normal steps in treating oral or nasal bleeding follow:

- Control hemorrhage
- Extract tooth, and close defect
- Prescribe postoperative antibiotics and manage pain
- Complete further diagnostics if not resolved

Stomatitis

Stomatitis is another condition that is generally chronic in nature, but acute flare-ups can make a patient very uncomfortable. Whether the problem is *CUPS* (chronic ulcerative paradental stomatitis) in a dog who exhibits highly painful "kissing ulcers" or lymphocytic/plasmacytic stomatitis (LPS) in a cat, these conditions can make patients so distraught that they stop eating completely. It is essential to schedule complete periodontal therapy to try to manage the condition, but you can provide more immediate relief with antibiotics, anti-inflammatories (if the condition is not viral in nature), and pain management. Once the condition is stabilized, many forms of treatment—from periodontal therapy with antibiotic perioceutics, local infiltration of anti-inflammatory drugs, and even extractions if necessary—can be steps in moderating the inflammation (see chapter 3: Periodontal Disease). Home care plays an important role in plaque control, but instruct the owners to be very careful in any attempts to handle pets with painful mouths!

Resorptive Lesions

Though primarily seen in cats, resorptive lesions can also occur in dogs, and in rare cases, they can have an acute presentation. Provide basic supportive therapy (antibiotics, pain management) until the lesions can be thoroughly evaluated radiographically and treated appropriately (see chapter 7: Feline Oral and Dental Diseases—Restorative).

Feline Oral and Dental Disease

Most of the preceding chapters dealt in general with both dogs and cats, though the majority of subjects covered were canine patients. Yet there are a number of distinct differences to be found in feline aspects of veterinary dentistry.

PERIODONTAL DISEASE IN CATS

The basic descriptions of the periodontal disease process and therapy were discussed in chapter 3, but specific aspects unique to feline periodontal disease are covered here.

Attachment

In cats, the sulcus depth is typically minimal, so any degree of pocket depth over 0.5 to 1.0 mm is considered abnormal and an indication of attachment loss. Add to that the diminutive size of some feline teeth and nearly any amount of attachment loss can endanger a tooth's integrity. This highlights the importance of preventing such loss, particularly in young animals with juvenile periodontitis. Some young cats with marked inflammation eventually "grow out" of the condition, so if attachment loss has been minimized with regular periodontal therapy and home care, many teeth can be preserved.

Chronic Periodontal Disease

Cats are also unique in their response to chronic, low-grade periodontal inflammation.

Chronic Alveolar Osteitis

This condition sometimes involves the mandibular symphysis region, and it is commonly associated with the maxillary canines. It produces a distinct bulging appearance of the osseous tissue at the rostral mandible or at the upper canines (Figure 7.1). Any suspicious tissue should, of course, be biopsied, but most cases of this nature are the result of chronic inflammation. Periodontal pockets may be present, and you should treat the teeth appropriately for any ongoing periodontal disease, but the chronic osseous changes are typically irreversible. At times, there will be sufficient inflammation and attachment loss to warrant extraction of the tooth, which generally is not too difficult. Closure of the extraction site can be very tricky, however, given the bulging alveolar bone and thin gingiva. Follow the basics steps of extraction to

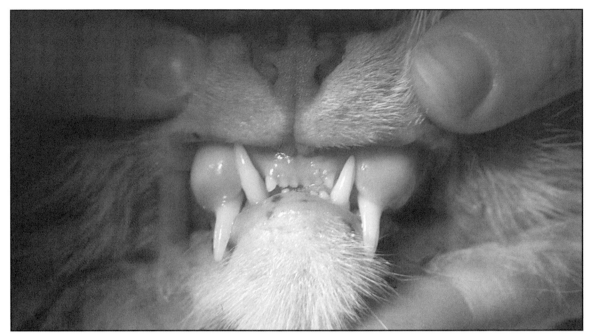

Figure 7.1 a *Bulging alveoli in a maxillary canine*

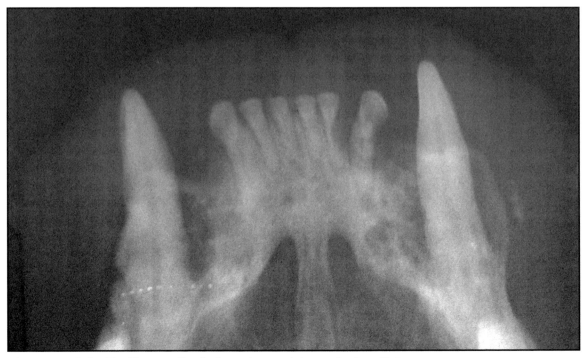

Figure 7.1 b *Radiograph of chronic osteitis and alveolitis*

make things go more smoothly: Make releasing incisions, raise a gingival flap while releasing connecting fibers under the mucogingival junction, and perform alveoloplasty to flatten the bulge.

Maxillary Canine Extrusion

In conjunction with chronic alveolitis or alone, cats can also manifest a unique response in which the maxillary canine teeth seem to "supererupt" or extrude (Figure 7.2). Whether the normal periodontal ligament forces exceed any counterforces of mastication or alveolar bone deposition at the apex works to "push" the tooth out, the effect is the same. The teeth can appear longer than normal, with increasing amounts of root exposure and sometimes trauma to the lower lip. If the tooth is stable, without periodontal pocket formation and with no radiographic signs of excessive bone loss, it can be preserved until attachment loss becomes significant. Gently blunt the tips of the elongated canine teeth (using a white stone bur on a high-speed handpiece with adequate water cooling) to minimize further lip trauma.

STOMATITIS

Among the most frustrating conditions involving feline mouths are the range of syndromes described by the term *stomatitis*. Varying degrees and regions of inflammation may be present, from marginal to hyperplastic gingivitis to palatitis to faucitis to having the entire oral cavity involved (Plates 17, 18, and 19).

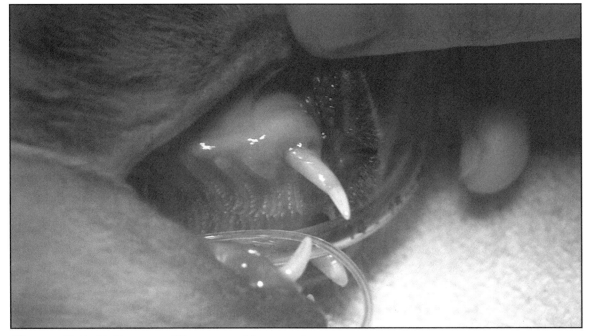

Figure 7.2 *Feline maxillary cuspid extrusion*

Immunological Basis

Lymphocytic-plasmacytic stomatitis may often be a histological diagnosis, reflective of the inflammatory cells utilized in an immune response. Some cats may exhibit stomatitis secondary to a deficient immune system resulting from viral infections such as feline leukemia virus (FeLV), feline immunosuppressive virus (FIV), calici virus, and others, but there are many patients with no demonstrable evidence of viral infection. With these patients, the probability exists that their immune systems are actually hyperresponsive to the bacteria present in plaque, a substance that is constantly present on teeth. Keeping a "plaque-intolerant" individual completely plaque free is nearly impossible, particularly if the animal's mouth is painful!

Therapy

The primary goal of treating chronic stomatitis is to minimize the inflammation in the first place by controlling the plaque. Although this is a rather idealistic goal, doing so can at least make some individuals more comfortable and can slow the disease progression. The use of antibiotics (though identifying a specific culture and sensitivity may not be too helpful) on an intermittent basis can help some individuals, as can doses of anti-inflammatory agents to suppress the overactive immune system. Many other therapies have been proposed and tried, with variable success, and new compounds are considered on a regular basis, some of which have had previous trials in the human field, such as CoQ-10.

In most individuals, the conservative therapy of dental cleanings, home care, antibiotics, and anti-inflammatories yields temporary benefits that diminish with time. As the condition worsens, the inflammation can cause significant oral pain and inappetence. To provide some relief in these patients, extraction of some or all of the caudal teeth (premolars and molars) may be necessary. Although this seems extreme to some, the degree of relief can be significant in many patients. It is vitally important to remove all tooth structure, leaving no root tips, and to smooth the alveolar bone before closure. If possible, it is best to leave the canine teeth, unless significant inflammation is present around them as well. If the stomatitis progresses to involve the canine teeth, they may eventually have to be extracted.

Even after extraction, particularly in chronic cases involving proliferative reaction in the *fauces* and pharyngeal regions, persistent inflammation can be present. Continued use of antibiotics and anti-inflammatory drugs (including intralesional injections of methylprednisolone) can be used to help control, though probably not cure, the inflammation.

RESORPTIVE LESIONS

No matter what you call feline dental resorptive lesions (cervical line lesions, neck lesions, feline odontoclastic resorptive lesions, etc.), these conditions are frustrating to manage (Table 7.1). To be sure, more is now known

Table 7.1
Resorptive lesions

Stage	Extent	Therapy
1	Into enamel	Debride, use liner, bonding agent, or fill
2	Into dentin	No root resorption—fill Root resorption—extract
3	Into pulp cavity	Extract (Rarely, use endodontics or restore)
4	Structural damage	Extract
5	Crown lost	Extract roots if inflamed, leave if healing

about histologic changes during their progression, but the exact causes of and influences on these lesions are still a mystery, though theories abound. From a practical standpoint, you need to know how to recognize and assess them and realize that they will often be progressive.

Signs

Resorptive lesions can be large enough to cause extensive crown loss that is immediately obvious, but often the initial lesions are hidden by calculus or hyperplastic gingiva that has grown into the lesion as an inflammatory response. These lesions may not always be apparent during an initial examination, so if a cat is presented for a dental cleaning, the owners should always leave a phone number at which they can be reached should lesions be found.

Whether the lesion is readily visible or covered with calculus and gingiva, cats will often exhibit a pain response or twitch when the lesion is touched during a routine cleaning, even with adequate levels of anesthesia. This discomfort can be present even in a shallow lesion, so such defects should never be overlooked. Premolars are frequently involved on the buccal surfaces, but molars, canines, and incisors, as well as all surfaces, are also susceptible.

One thing is certain with resorptive lesions: Complete assessment, including intraoral radiology, is necessary to determine the extent of the lesion. No matter how minor the external appearance might be, you must keep in mind the potential for root resorption (internal or external) that may also extend into the crown (Figure 7.3).

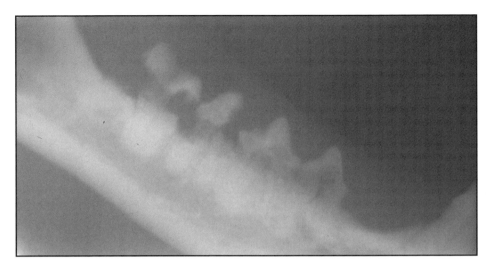

Figure 7.3
Radiograph of multiple resorptive lesions with root involvement

Stages

Determining the stage of the lesion will help you plan the appropriate treatment. A dental explorer (the shepherd's hook at the opposite end of most periodontal probes) is an important tactile tool to use in looking for *erosions* (Figure 7.4). In addition to identifying the larger cavitations, you should use the sharp explorer tip, gently feeling for any defect or roughness along the cervical (neck) region of the teeth, particularly in furcations. If there is an irregularity, the tip will hang up or catch in the erosive defect. Once a lesion is identified, determine the extent of involvement with a combination of visual, tactile, and radiographic assessment.

Stage 1

The earliest stage of resorptive lesions involves the enamel only. Lesions are seldom caught this early, though you may identify a roughened area at a furcation or minor defects. Even at this stage, you should take radiographs, and if a minor lesion is present, teeth will have solid roots with distinct periodontal ligament space and canals.

Stage 2

Once some of the dentin has been lost, a distinct defect should be identifiable. This is probably the most important stage to assess fully because even a fairly well-contained coronal lesion can exhibit significant levels of external and internal root resorption radiographically.

Stage 3

Extension of the defect into the *pulp cavity* immediately worsens the prognosis for the tooth. Any indication of pulpal bleeding warrants a specific assessment of the canal system radiographically. It is rare to find an unaffected pulp cavity in such a lesion.

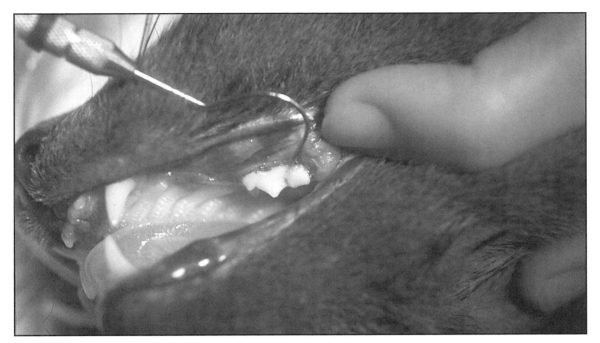

Figure 7.4 *Periodontal explorer in resorptive lesion*

Stage 4

Left unchecked, resorptive lesions can progress past *pulpal exposure* to the point at which extensive structural crown damage is present (Figure 7.5). Frequently, extensive resorption of the roots is also seen.

Stage 5

With sufficient structural damage, the crown will eventually be lost, often leaving some root structure subgingivally. In some cases, the gingiva will heal without inflammation at the site, as the odontoclastic resorption continues to resorb the roots, with eventual conversion to osseous tissue. It is almost as if the body were trying to resolve the situation on its own.

Treatment

No matter what level of involvement is encountered or which therapy is selected, you must always inform the owners that this disease tends to be progressive. This prepares them for the possibility of early lesions worsening (even with fillings) or the development of new lesions, which would become apparent during subsequent visits.

Stage 1

If you do encounter the very shallow stage 1 lesions or even suspicious areas of mild furcation exposure that have a rougher surface, there is some indication

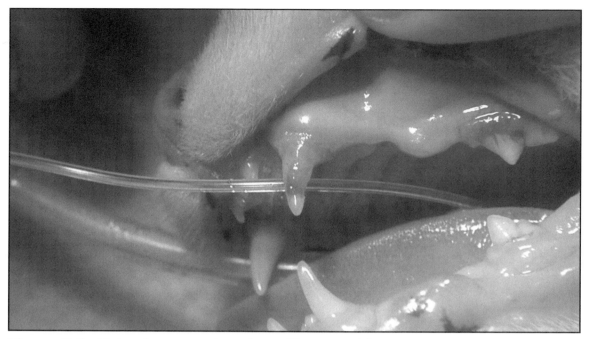

Figure 7.5 *Extensive resorption of maxillary cuspid*

that you should consider treating the lesion to hopefully interrupt the progression, provided the roots look normal on radiographs. Gently debride the area to remove any inflammatory components, whether to excise hyperplastic gingiva or to curette odontoclastic cells from the tooth surface or adjacent alveolar bone. You can carefully use a periodontal curette or a white stone bur on a high-speed handpiece with water coolant. Polish the surface with a nonfluoride pumice (flour pumice), and control hemorrhage in the area. If the area is just roughened enamel, place a fluoride *varnish* and allow it to dry, or use a dentinal bonding agent. Several filling products can be used in filling erosive lesions, including *glass ionomers* that bond directly to dentin and even release fluoride. This is preferable over other restorative agents that might require removal of some of the tooth for mechanical retention, which you should avoid. Newer composites, including some glass ionomer–composite combinations or flowable products, can have sufficient retention through the use of bonding agents. Because these lesions are seldom found on high-stress areas, these products are usually adequate. There is some level of technique sensitivity to each product, so become familiar with the material of your choice (see chapter 9: Materials and Equipment). With restorative placement, the margins should be smooth, and there should be no overfill or underfill.

Stage 2

The first step in treating a stage 2 lesion is to decide whether to restore or extract the tooth. The importance of radiographs cannot be overemphasized because many relatively innocuous-looking lesions can have significant root resorption, which would be a contraindication for restoration. Even if the roots look great, however, you need to tell the owner that additional progression is possible after the restoration is placed.

Under optimal conditions (distinct shallow lesion with good root structure and good follow-up plan), some teeth may be amenable to filling, particularly if the client is well informed and wishes to try to preserve the tooth. In addition, with a more "strategic" tooth (canines, upper fourth premolars, lower first molars), preservation should be considered if there is a chance of at least prolonging the tooth's function while also providing pain relief.

Prepare the area as outlined before, debriding and providing hemostasis. If the defect gets close to or extends into the subgingival area, you should raise a flap to expose the area (envelope or flap with releasing incisions). Curette the adjacent alveolar bone to get clean margins. Once the lesion is prepped, you should place the restorative following the manufacturer's directions and finish the margins (see chapter 5: Advanced Oral and Dental Problems, especially the section on restoratives), closing the flap if necessary. Anytime lesions are encountered, you should recommend a regular home-care regimen and routine dental rechecks and therapy.

Advanced Lesions (Stages 3 to 5)

Once the canal is exposed, there are only rare occasions on which restoration is warranted. For example, if a canine tooth has canal exposure but no further indication of root resorption (internal or external), a full standard endodontics procedure (root canal) with restoration may be considered. For the vast majority of affected teeth, however, extraction is by far the treatment of choice.

Making the decision to extract, though, is often easier than the extraction itself. With the resorption that is frequently present, the roots tend to be both fragile and nearly ankylosed to the alveolar bone. Again, radiographs are extremely important in preextraction assessment. Even if faced with abnormal-looking roots, you should still follow a systematic approach to extraction: making a gingival flap, sectioning, removing alveolar bone, and elevating (see chapter 4: Oral Surgery—Extraction). Smaller, more delicate elevators that have a sharpened working end that cups the root structure will give you more control (see chapter 9: Materials and Equipment). If there was not a distinct periodontal ligament space present, chances are the tooth won't elevate easily as in a routine extraction. In fact, breaking the crown or root or having it crumble completely is not uncommon. Certainly, if the root does start to loosen, elevate it if at all possible. If the root does fracture, you should make every reasonable attempt to extract the remaining tooth structure, including moderate alveolar bone removal and elevation. Pulverization of the root tips (using a round bur on a high-speed handpiece) is a possible means of removing them, but unless this procedure can be well monitored with radiographs and performed with reasonable skill, you should not attempt it.

In some teeth, roots can resorb, becoming ankylosed and even converted into osseous tissue, and attempts at complete extraction could compromise the jaw structure and strength. If this is the case and if elevation has not been effective, you may consider removing as much tooth as possible (crown and neck) without damaging the jaw. What remains of the root(s) will likely continue to be resorbed and be remodeled into bone. This procedure must be accompanied by a radiograph, noted in the records, and discussed with the owner, with radiographic follow-up done to ensure there are no future complications at the site. Optimally, you should place an *osseoconductive* material into the extraction site before suturing to stimulate complete bony healing in the region. One situation in which this procedure would not be acceptable would be a case of stomatitis, where all tooth and root structure must be removed to avoid any continued antigenic stimulation.

SQUAMOUS CELL CARCINOMA

In cats, squamous cell carcinoma (SCC) is the most common malignancy in the oral cavity (see chapter 2: Oral Examination and Recognition of Pathology—Tumors). Tonsillar forms are very aggressive and metastasize early, and sublingual forms with extensive local infiltration are difficult to resect completely without damaging vital structures. SCC found in the mandible, however, can sometimes be managed by removal of the affected mandible (hemimandibulectomy) (Figure 7.6). Although this may seem a rather aggressive approach, most patients tolerate it fairly well, usually adjusting to

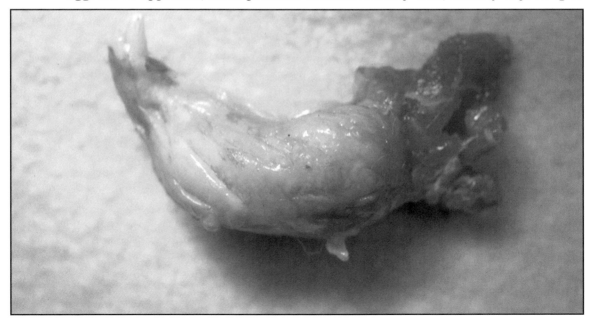

Figure 7.6 *Feline mandible with squamous cell carcinoma after hemimandibulectomy*

the drift of the other mandible. The procedure itself isn't excessively difficult, and it is covered in numerous surgical texts. You can also use this procedure in cases with extensive damage to a mandible (because of fracture, gunshot, etc.). Postoperative care includes supportive care, particularly if the appetite is disrupted (i.e., tube feeding).

EOSINOPHILIC GRANULOMA COMPLEX

Although the lesions in this syndrome are not neoplastic, at times this must be confirmed by biopsy. Whether rodent (indolent) ulcers on the lip (Figure 7.7), eosinophilic plaques, or even linear granulomas, the potential immune-related biological activity of these lesions often make them amenable to anti-inflammatory therapy.

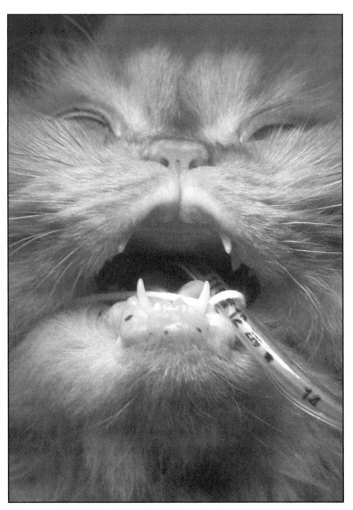

Figure 7.7 *Rodent (indolent) ulcer on upper lips*

CHAPTER 8

Oral and Dental Disease in Pocket Pets

With today's hectic lifestyles and more people living in cramped quarters, smaller pets requiring less routine daily care are becoming more popular. Increasingly, chinchillas, hamsters, gerbils, guinea pigs, rabbits, ferrets and other small animals have become household pets, and along with this trend has come a host of special dental problems for you to address. This chapter will deal with some of the more common dental problems of these unique pets and how to handle them.

TOOTH ANATOMY

You must first become acquainted with the general dental anatomy of three groups of pocket pets: rodents, lagomorphs, and carnivores. Within these groups, you will find both *aradicular hypsodont* and *brachyodont* teeth.

An aradicular hypsodont tooth is one that has no true root but only a crown, some of which is submerged. These teeth will continue to grow throughout the animal's and the tooth's life. For this reason, the periodontal ligament has an intermediate plexus attachment between the alveolar bone and the tooth to allow continued tooth eruption without destroying the periodontal ligament. These teeth must be worn down by attrition or wear to the teeth from mastication. Failure to have proper wear leads to dental, oral, and physical disease for these pets. Aradicular hypsodont incisors have enamel covering the front and sides but not the back or top of the tooth. This specialized enamel on the front of the incisor teeth commonly takes on a yellow to deep-orange color (Figure 8.1).

Brachyodont teeth have both a crown and a true root structure. These teeth are complete upon eruption; they do not continue to grow or erupt, and they are not meant to wear down continuously as do the hypsodont teeth. The crowns of brachyodont teeth are normally completely covered with enamel of various shades of white.

DENTAL FORMULAS

The specific numbers of the different tooth types (incisors, canines, premolars, molars) can help group an animal into a species category. A primary difference between lagomorphs and rodents is that rodents have one pair of maxillary incisors whereas lagomorphs have a second pair of smaller peg

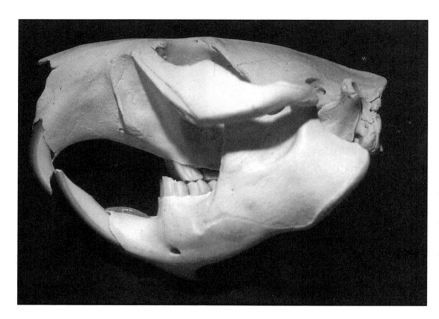

Figure 8.1
Beaver skull showing dark enamel on incisors and chisel edges

incisors behind the larger first pair (Figure 8.2).

Rodents

The rodents have more dental variation. They, like the lagomorphs, have incisors, premolars, and molars but no canine teeth. In addition, some in this group, such as the guinea pig and the chinchilla, have both incisors and cheek teeth that continually grow. Others, such as mice, rats, and hamsters, have continually growing incisors (aradicular hypsodont teeth), but their cheek teeth (premolars and molars) are brachyodonts that do not continue to grow.

The dental formulas of hamsters, Old World mice and rats, mice and rats, gerbils, and guinea pigs and chinchillas are written as follows:

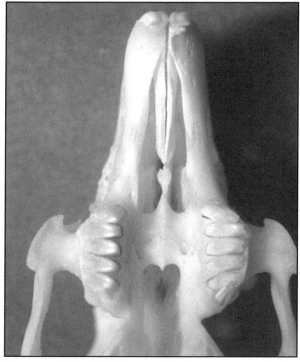

Figure 8.2 *Rabbit maxilla, large upper incisor pair with smaller peg incisors behind and large diastema between incisors and cheek teeth*

Hamsters   2 × (I 1/1, C 0/0, PM 0/0, M 23/23) = 12 to 16 total teeth
Old World mice and rats (*Muridae*)
            2 × (I 1/1, C 0/0, PM 0/0, M 23/23) = 12 to 16 total teeth
Mice and rats (*Cricetidae*)
            2 × (I 1/1, C 0/0, PM 0/0, M 3/3) = 16 total teeth
Gerbils   2 × (I 1/1, C 0/0, PM 0/0, M 3/3) = 16 total teeth
Guinea pigs and chinchillas
            2 × (I 1/1, C 0/0, PM 1/1, M 3/3) = 20 total teeth
Squirrels   2 × (I 1/1, C 0/0, PM 12/1, M 3/3) = 20 to 22 total teeth

Lagomorphs

The lagomorphs (rabbits, hares, cottontails, pikas, etc.) have aradicular hypsodont teeth, both in the anterior teeth (incisors) and cheek teeth (premolar and molars); they have no canine teeth.

The dental formulas of rabbits, hares, and squirrels are written as follows:

Rabbit   2 × (I 2/1, C 0/0, PM 3/2, M 23/3) = 26 to 28 total teeth
Hare   2 × (I 2/1, C 0/0, PM 3/2, M 3/3) = 28 total teeth

Carnivores

The carnivores, by contrast, have only brachyodont teeth, which are somewhat similar to the dog and cat teeth that you are probably more familiar with. They have incisors, canines, premolars, and molars. The most common exotic small pet within this group is the ferret.

The dental formula of the ferret is written as follows:

Ferret   2 × (I 3/3, C 1/1, PM 3/3, M 1/2) = 34 total teeth

ORAL EXAMINATION

The oral examination of a pocket pet usually consists of two parts: a survey of a conscious patient and a more complete examination with sedation. Most domesticated ferrets, with their carnivore teeth and occlusion, have mouths that can be opened fairly widely for initial evaluation. Rodents and lagomorphs have small mouths and a temporomandibular joint (TMJ) that greatly limits the opening of the mouth, so it is more difficult to get a good survey oral examination without sedation. Many of these small pets can be restrained relatively well by simply wrapping a towel around the body, leaving the head exposed for the examination.

You can examine the anterior (incisor and canine) teeth with the aid of a good light and a little gentle coaxing to open the mouth. Magnification can also be of great help, and a good otoscope and ear cone can often allow a reasonable oral exam, not only of the posterior teeth but also of the cheeks, palate, and tongue. Radiographs can be of an immense aid in diagnosing many elusive oral conditions. A nasoscope or an endoscope can also be of value in the oral examination.

When the pet is sedated, the use of mouth gags, cheek retractors, tongue retractors, good lighting, and magnification can greatly improve your visualization of the inside of the oral cavity (Figure 8.3). Intraoral films (sizes #0 to #2) can often be used in the mouth for true intraoral radiographs, and size #4 intraoral dental film can be used for diagnostic extraoral views. Careful palpation of the jaws and face may give indications as to the location of developing pathology, and you can manipulate the jaws in a chewing motion to identify any limits or restrictions of the occlusal movements.

ANESTHESIA

You can use both injectables and inhalants in dental procedures, but the safety and quick recovery from inhalants such as isoflurane make them the preferred anesthesia for most dental cases.

Rodents and Lagomorphs

In the rodents and lagomorphs, inhalant anesthesia for dental treatment is initially administered by induction in a chamber, then if intubation is not possible, it is maintained with intermittent masking. Intubation is by far the better approach, but the technique can sometimes be difficult to learn. The pediatric laryngoscope, an otoscope with a long ear cone, and an endoscope can

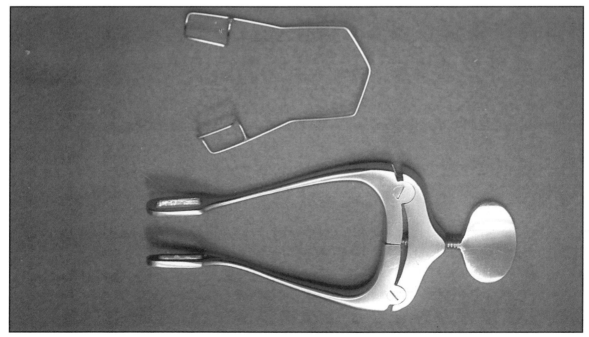

Figure 8.3 *Mouth gags and retractors*

all be helpful in visualization for intubation. Laryngeal spasms can usually be decreased by the light topical use of a 4% lidocaine solution. Small endotracheal tubes, varying in size from 2.0 to 4.0 mm (ID), are used for most of rabbits, guinea pigs, and chinchillas. However, for hamsters, gerbils, mice, and rats, size 12- to 20-gauge intravenous (IV) catheters with the stylet removed may be used, but they can be difficult to connect to an anesthesia machine without creative work on the connections.

Ferrets

In the ferret, masking or placing the animal in an anesthesia chamber is typically the most satisfactory mode of induction. These animals appear to tolerate isoflurane very well. Once the animal is well sedated, a size 2.0 to 5.0 mm (ID) endotracheal tube can be passed and secured with umbilical tape or a rubber band.

Monitoring Anesthesia

Having an alert technician is one of the best ways to ensure the monitoring of these delicate small pets. However, a good pulse oximeter can provide an additional level of assessment. Because the small tubes are easily clogged by mucous and other debris, check their patency every 2 to 3 minutes, and keep spare tubes for quick replacement close at hand. The regular endotracheal tubes can often be kept clear with a cotton swab or the use of a feline tomcat catheter on a syringe to provide suction for mucous and debris removal.

CHARTING

All pathology should be recorded or charted. The use of specialized charts can be very helpful, but such charts are not absolutely required.

ORAL DISEASES AND THEIR TREATMENTS

There are many oral and dental diseases of the small pocket pets. In this section, we will discuss some of the more common, along with possible treatments.

Gingivitis

Gingivitis, an inflammation of the gingiva, is typically initiated in rodents and lagomorphs by rough edges on food and watering devices. Have the owner remove or replace the offending device. Once this is accomplished, healing is usually rapid. You can place a few coats of tincture of myrrh and benzoin or apply an oral antiseptic solution when needed.

In ferrets, gingivitis is more commonly caused by bacterial plaque activity, and if untreated, it may progress into periodontal disease. Treatment is generally a good oral hygiene program at home. The use of oral antiseptic solutions may help in control, but brushing the teeth with an edible toothpaste made for animals is one of the most effective ways to remove the plaque film from the teeth.

Periodontal Disease

Periodontal disease is an infection of the periodontal tissues: gums, periodontal ligament, cementum, or alveolar bone. It results in the gradual loss of the tooth's supporting periodontium and eventually possibly the tooth itself. Periodontal disease will commonly form around brachyodont teeth (in ferrets and some rodents), but lagomorph teeth or rodent incisors are less likely to develop periodontal problems. Treatment is a combination of routine professional teeth cleaning and a good oral hygiene program at home.

Cheek Pouch Impaction

Cheek pouch impaction sometimes occurs in rodents and lagomorphs when food is packed into the cheek pouch and becomes doughy or dry and the animal cannot loosen and remove it. An inflammation or infection may develop in the soft tissues surrounding the material itself, or bacterial by-products can irritate the tissues. Treatment consists of removing the food and applying an oral antiseptic.

Stomatitis

Stomatitis in rodents and lagomorphs is most commonly a condition secondary to food impactions or vitamin C deficiencies (in guinea pigs), resulting in a scurvy problem. Treatment includes immediate therapy with vitamin C supplements, correction of the dietary deficiency that caused the problem, and supportive care, such as fluids and possibly tube feeding. Vitamin C in foods is gradually depleted by oxidation. For this reason, most manufacturers of rodent diets, such as those for the guinea pigs, date the food so an owner will know when it needs to be replaced.

Slobbers or Wet Dewlap

Slobbers or wet dewlap is a secondary problem caused by excessive salivation, secondarily due to some form of oral or dental problem that may lead to an infection of the skin in the hair around the lower face or dewlap in lagomorphs and rodents. Treatment involves finding and treating the initiating cause of the excessive salivation. You must also treat the skin infection by clipping the hair in the area of infection for good hygiene. The area must be cleansed and treated with antiseptic solutions or antibiotics.

Enamel Hypocalcification (Hypoplasia)

Enamel hypocalcification or hypoplasia refers to an area on the tooth that is undermineralized, weak, and maybe chalky white or discolored brown. In the continually growing teeth in the lagomorphs and rodents, no treatment for such a lesion is usually required. The lesion is only a temporary problem in most cases because it is eventually lost as tooth eruption and wear removes it. However, if such lesions are seen on a regular basis, the food and water sources and the animal's general health should be examined to determine the underlying cause and resolve it. High fluoride levels in the food or water can cause these lesions, as can infections or high fevers and certain other diseases. In the ferret, however, the lesions are of a permanent nature. Small lesions may be cleaned, and diseased enamel can be lightly scrubbed away using a high-speed handpiece and then sealing the dentin with several coats of dentinal bonding agent and possibly some composite restorative work.

Tooth Caries

Tooth caries or bacterial-related cavities are rarely seen among pocket pets and occur only in the brachyodont cheek teeth in rodents and the cheek teeth in the ferret. When they do occur, they may be seen on the crown or on the root surfaces, where they can be difficult to detect. Generally, extraction is the treatment of choice for most of the rodents, as the lesions are typically advanced before they are detected. In the ferret, if the lesions are caught early enough, they can be treated by removal of all decay and the placement of a composite or glass ionomer filling. However, if the lesions are extensive, extraction may be the only alternative. When lesions are found, the application of fluoride to the teeth may reduce future occurrences.

Fractured Teeth

Fractured teeth must be dealt with on an individual basis. In the ferret and rodent brachyodont teeth, the options are basically endodontics, such as a root canal, or extraction. In the rodent's and lagomorph's continually growing teeth, pulp capping is generally the first choice because extraction may lead to malocclusions of the opposing teeth that may then grow excessively long without the attritional wear provided by the extracted tooth. If extraction is required, it must be understood that these malocclusions may develop and need continued observation and treatment by floating or odontoplasty.

Abscessed Teeth

Abscessed teeth can develop from either periodontal or endodontic diseases. In most cases, extraction is the treatment of choice. The actual abscess may require incision, drainage, and cleansing. Antibiotics may be appropriate, but extreme caution should be used in their selection and use.

Antibiotic Caution: Many lagomorphs and rodents are highly sensitive to some antibiotics. Their use can lead to fatal enteritis complications on occasion. Chloramphenicol is generally the drug of choice for the treatment of enteropathy conditions. Supportive care may also be required.

Tongue Tied

Tongue tied in most rodent and lagomorph cases is a condition in which usually the lower teeth overgrow and actually pin the tongue to the roof of the mouth. The associated trauma, inflammation, and infection can easily lead to death. Treatment normally consists of cutting the overgrown teeth with molar or bone cutters to release the tongue. In addition, antibiotics, anti-inflammatories, fluids, and other supportive care may be required. Once this condition occurs, a poor long-term prognosis should be given because the problem has a tendency to recur. Prevention normally includes close observation and floating of the teeth as needed.

Malocclusions

Malocclusions are typically divided into two types: traumatic and *atraumatic malocclusions.*

Traumatic Malocclusions

Traumatic malocclusions result from traumatic injuries to the teeth that cause the loss of a portion of the crown and the loss of the occlusal contacts and normal wear of the opposing tooth. Two items must be addressed and treated in this regard: the injury to the traumatized tooth and the overgrowth of the opposing tooth. Smooth the jagged edges of the traumatized tooth to reduce soft-tissue injuries. If the pulp chamber has been opened and the pulp exposed, perform a pulp capping and filling. A small amount of calcium hydroxide placed over the exposed pulp and a glass ionomer filling placed to protect the endodontic system may help to maintain the tooth's vitality. The opposing tooth should have routine odontoplasty performed in order to prevent excessive overgrowth and soft-tissue injuries until the traumatized tooth has grown to once again become interactive with the occlusion of the opposing tooth.

Atraumatic Malocclusions

Atraumatic malocclusions are those not attributed to a traumatic injury. These are normally the result of some form of nutritional problem that has resulted in poor growth or weakness in the jaws or hereditary conditions resulting in malocclusion of the teeth. Generally, these can be further divided into four categories: atraumatic anterior malocclusions, atraumatic posterior malocclusions, dietary malocclusions, and behavioral malocclusions.

Atraumatic Anterior Malocclusions. These malocclusions are genetically caused by a short maxillary diastema, resulting in a malocclusion and overgrowth of the incisor teeth. This condition typically expresses itself within the first year of life. The prognosis is good with either routine odontoplasty of the incisor teeth or their extraction.

Atraumatic Posterior Malocclusions. These malocclusions are caused by some shift in the mandibular occlusion. This shift may result from nutritional deficiencies, genetic predisposition, or other physiologic action working on the stability of the mandibular occlusion. This action may work upon the mandibular symphysis, body, or TMJ to result is the pathological shift. These malocclusions more normally demonstrate themselves after 2 years of age and carry a poor long-term prognosis because of the secondary health problems that commonly develop. Always inform the owner of the poor prognosis, even when the patient appears to be in good condition at the time of diagnosis. It is not uncommon for this condition to result in a secondary malocclusion of the incisor teeth, which occurs later in life than a primary anterior malocclusion. Antibiotics, anti-inflammatories, pain control medications, and fluids will be indicated at times. The owner should be educated about providing supportive care—keeping the animal comfortable, warm, hydrated and hand feeding of a soft diet to maintain reasonable nutritional intake. Should the pet become depressed or be in constant discomfort, euthanasia should be considered.

Atraumatic Dietary Malocclusions. These malocclusions result from an improper diet that fails to provide the required attritional wear to the teeth. Dietary problems are easily corrected by providing the proper diet for the pet and performing temporary odontoplasty or floating of the teeth until the dietary correction has time to provide a natural rectification of the problem.

Atraumatic Behavioral Malocclusions. These malocclusions result from behavioral problems of cribbing, barbering, or other improper chewing activity. These are typically a result of some form of anxiety or neurosis in the pet. Treatment involves not only odontoplasty or floating of teeth but also the removal of the pet's stress factors, but this can be complex, as the cause of the anxiety or neurosis often is not be readily apparent. In some cases, moving the cage, adding or removing a companion pet, enlarging the cage, or adding toys, mazes, or other items to occupy the animal's time may help, but these cases can sometimes be frustrating to treat.

Incisor Overgrowth

Incisor overgrowth is easily treated when not complicated by cheek tooth involvement. Treatment selection may be guided by the severity of the problem, its chronicity, the lack of opposing tooth interaction, and client preference. Ordinarily, there are two choices: odontoplasty to reconfigure the teeth in hopes of reestablishing a normal functional occlusion, or extraction. In many cases, if one incisor must be extracted, eventually all four may have to follow suit or routine odontoplasty must be performed to maintain a functional occlusion.

Cheek Tooth Overgrowth

This condition almost always has a poor long-term prognosis. The overgrowth cannot be well controlled because of the animal's restrictive anatomy and the fact that the condition is usually well advanced before being discovered (Figure 8.4). The chronic nature of the disease and associated inflammation and infection result in many serious secondary health problems. Treatment consists

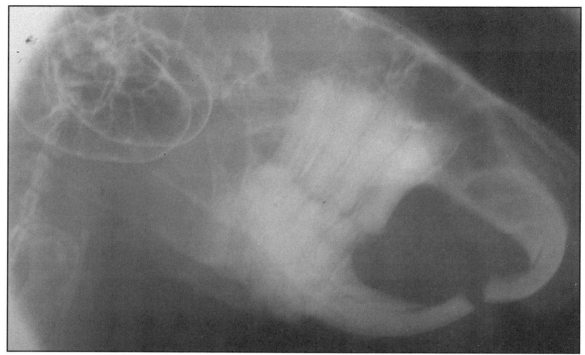

Figure 8.4 *Radiograph of chinchilla with cheek teeth overgrowth*

of routine floating of the teeth, use of antibiotics and anti-inflammatories, and supportive therapies such as fluids, hand or tube feeding, pain medications, and maintenance of a reasonable body temperature.

TREATMENT

The same treatments may apply for several conditions, whether it's regular crown reduction for maintenance or extraction. Supportive care can be crucial in keeping the patient healthy.

Floating or Odontoplasty

Floating or odontoplasty is the filing down of the teeth if they grow unchecked. In the anterior teeth (incisors), this can be done with a crosscut bur or white stone abrasive point used on a high- or low-speed dental handpiece very effectively. The cheek teeth in the posterior of the mouth can be more difficult to safely reach with the dental handpieces and burs. In the posterior cheek teeth (premolars and molars), floats that are files or rasps with a handle are commonly used to remove excess tooth structure (Figure 8.5). These hand floats are not as efficient or as rapid as the burs used in the incisor teeth. Bone files and rasps are commonly used as dental floats in many of these cases.

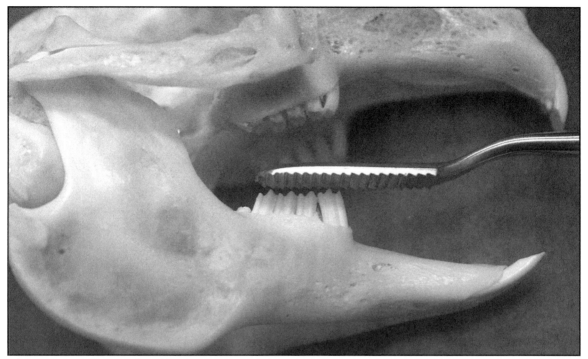

Figure 8.5 *Example of how a rasp can be used for odontoplasty (easier on a skull than on a patient!)*

Extractions in Rodents and Lagomorphs

Extractions in rodents and lagomorphs can be done with several different tools. The exact instruments vary with the tooth location and the size of the pet. When possible, extraction sites should be sutured closed. In addition, in order to help maintain the strength of the mandible, it is best to pack the extraction site before closure with a product such as Consil (Nutramax Labs, Baltimore, MD 21236) that will aid in promoting bone growth into the vacated tooth socket.

The anterior teeth (incisors) are held in place by the periodontal ligament. Because these teeth are continually growing, the periodontal ligament has an intermediate plexus that allows the tooth eruption movement. This means the ligament can be fairly easily broken down with proper elevation for tooth extraction. Most of the holding power of the periodontal ligament in these teeth is in the upper third of the submerged portion of the tooth. A No.1 or No.2 Winged Elevator (DentalAire, Fountain Valley, CA 92708), a Crossley Rabbit Luxator (Jorgensen Labs, Loveland, CO 80538), or even a blunted 18- to 20-gauge needle can be used to elevate these teeth. Once loosened, grasp the tooth with small extraction forceps, and gently pull it, keeping in mind its long archlike shape.

Removing the posterior teeth can be more difficult. If they are diseased to the point of being loose, they can be grasped with a 90° angle small forceps and removed. Other cheek teeth may need to be repelled, which requires a surgical approach to the root of the tooth.

CHAPTER 9

Materials and Equipment

As veterinary dentistry has evolved, so has the veterinary dentist's armamentarium. Many of the materials and pieces of equipment utilized by the veterinary dentist is the same or similar to that found in human dentistry, with some exceptions and adaptations to allow for variations in species. The materials and equipment covered in this section deal primarily with periodontics, oral surgery, radiography, operative or restorative dentistry, and endodontics. If you are just starting out, the most essential equipment to acquire, other than implements used for scaling and polishing, will be the periodontal probe, periodontal curettes, a means to take intraoral radiographs, a periosteal elevator, and some method of sectioning teeth and removing bone for extractions (Figure 9.1).

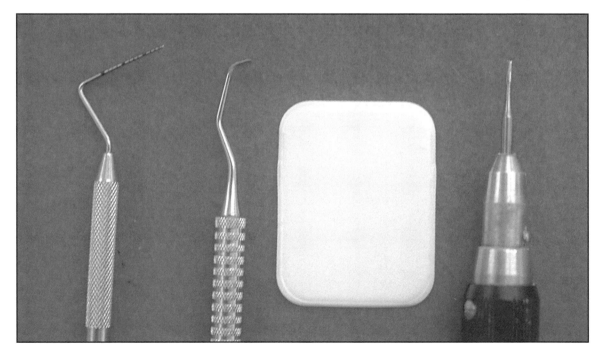

Figure 9.1 *Essentials for dental practice: Periodontal probe, curette, intraoral radiograph, means of sectioning teeth and removing alveolar bone (periosteal elevator not pictured)*

PERIODONTAL INSTRUMENTS

Periodontal disease and therapy constitute a significant portion of the veterinary dentist's caseload. The instrumentation is equally important for accurate diagnosis and proper treatment. The instruments are generally classified as hand instruments, power equipment, and instruments for prophylaxis or home care.

Hand Instruments

Of the hand instruments, the tool of choice for diagnosing periodontal disease is the periodontal probe. This handpiece has an angled tip and blunt end, with measurements in 1- to 3-mm increments or colors that allow for assessment of the depth of the gingival sulcus around the teeth. In general, periodontal probe depths greater than 3 to 4 mm in the dog and 0.5 mm in the cat are considered abnormal and should be further investigated by visual exam or radiography. The explorer is a thin, sharp-pointed instrument often placed on the opposite end of the periodontal probe as a shepherd's hook (Figure 9.2). This tactile-sensitive tool is used to detect pits in enamel, fissures, "sticky" cavitations, open endodontic canals, and dental resorptive lesions. Used together, these tools—the probe and the explorer—detect much of the periodontal problems encountered in veterinary dentistry.

Hand instruments can also be utilized for periodontal treatment. Plaque and calculus contribute to periodontal disease and should be removed both above and below the gumline. A pair of dental or tartar forceps can initially be

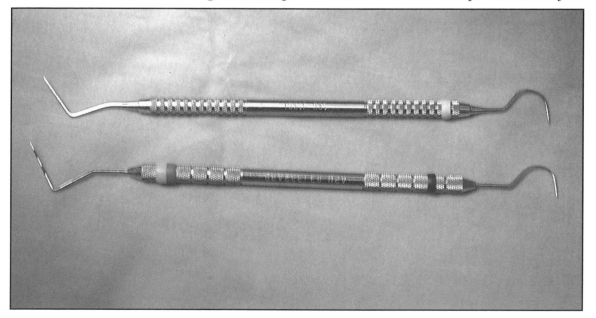

Figure 9.2 *Periodontal probe-explorer*

used to carefully remove large chunks of calculus before proceeding. You can use a sickle scaler to remove supragingival calculus (the calculus seen above the gumline). The sickle scaler has two cutting edges and is angled sharply on the back, creating a triangle shape in cross section of the working end. The scaler is not recommended for calculus removal below the gumline due to the angulation on the back and the sharp tip, which could damage the gingival attachment if pushed into the gingival sulcus. For removal of subgingival calculus (that calculus along the crown and root below the gumline), the curette is the instrument of choice. Curettes have one or two cutting edges, but unlike the scaler, they have a rounded back on the working end, forming a half-moon shape on cross section. This allows the toe to be gently placed below the gingival margin into the sulcus, or periodontal pocket, with less damage to the tissue. Universal curettes have two cutting edges with an 80° to 90° blade angulation to the shaft, and the shaft is angled to the handle to allow a 45–90° orientation of the blade against the tooth when the handle is parallel to the working surface. With such angles, only one of the cutting edges is typically effective for a particular tooth surface. The curette is a double-ended instrument, with working ends that are mirror images, adapted to allow proper instrumentation of all tooth surfaces. Each area-specific curette, such as the Gracey curette, was developed for a particular area or even a specific tooth surface in the human oral cavity, with an offset blade and only one cutting edge.

Using pull strokes, you can remove the calculus from the tooth surface until smooth. Curettes also can be used to gently debride the internal gingival surface of the sulcus to remove necrotic tissue and bacteria. This process is called subgingival curettage. Scalers and curettes are very effective for the removal of calculus, but these instruments also can be slow and fatiguing to use for the operator if large amounts of calculus are encountered. To minimize operator fatigue, proper use of the instrument includes use of a Modified Pen Grasp. With this, you grasp the instrument handle between the thumb and index finger and place the middle finger on the shaft near the working head. Place your ring finger on a tooth surface or nearby structure to provide stability and to act as a fulcrum. A wrist motion of activation with rotation of the wrist is more efficient and less fatiguing than a digital motion.

Hand instruments can become dull over time and will periodically need sharpening, which enhances effectiveness and prolongs their usefulness. Sharpening technique is a learned skill, and there are many manuals that detail it well (e.g., dental hygiene texts, manufacturer's booklets). You can use a conical stone to sharpen the face of the instrument during a procedure, but this method wears down the instrument more rapidly. A lightly oiled, flat Arkansas stone is best to sharpen cutting edges at approximately a 70° to 80° angle to the stone, matching the contour of the blade. Move the instrument back and forth on the stone in short strokes, starting near the portion of the head closest to the shank and advancing toward the toe or tip. Use a conical stone in a light stroking action to smooth any rough edges.

Power Instruments

Power instrumentation also is an effective means of calculus removal and can provide assistance in many other aspects of veterinary dentistry, as well. In practices that offer substantial dental services, the benefit of having an air-driven dental unit with compressor can be significant (Figure 9.3). With such power available, whether in the form of a small, "silent," chairside compressor or a larger remote one, the variety of handpieces available can facilitate any task.

A high-speed handpiece can accommodate any number of burs for sectioning teeth, drilling cavity preparations or endodontic access, finishing restoratives, and even performing gingivectomies with water irrigation (Figure 9.4). The high-speed port can also be used for a *sonic scaler* handpiece. The low-speed handpiece is primarily used for polishing angles, but reduction-angle gears and *straight handpieces* have multiple uses with the low-speed port as well (Figure 9.5). The air-water syringe, though not absolutely necessary for a dental practice, certainly can make things easier by providing handy irrigation, rinsing, and air drying.

Not every clinic will have such a unit, particularly if dentistry services are just being introduced. It is vital, however, to be able to perform some of the functions, most importantly those using burs for tooth sectioning and alveoloplasty. Simple units such as a Dremel tool (Dremel, Racine, WI) utilize straight handpiece burs that can perform these tasks, but speed control is sometimes not accurate; moreover, an external source of water for cooling and irrigation is

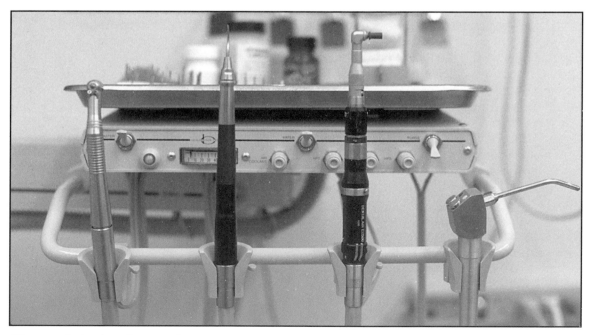

Figure 9.3 *Air-driven dental unit with (from left to right) high-speed handpiece with bur, sonic scaler, low-speed handpiece with prophy angle, air-water syringe*

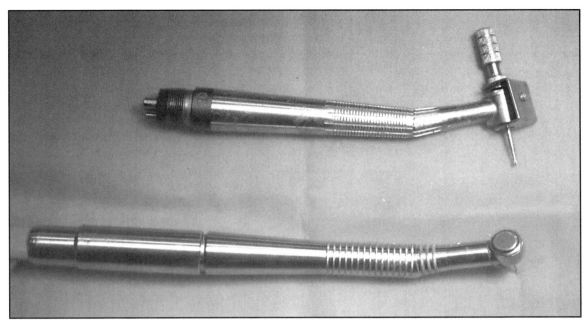

Figure 9.4 *High-speed handpiece, with automatic bur release or chuck release*

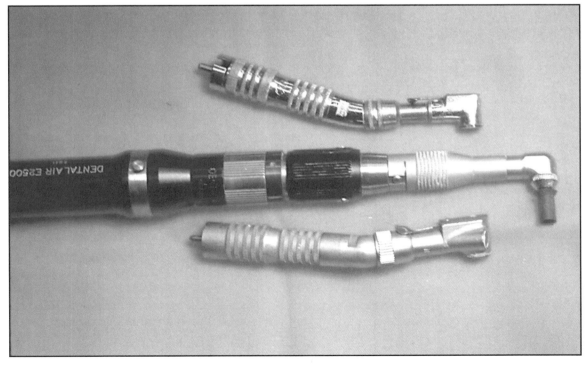

Figure 9.5 *Low-speed handpiece, with prophy angle and reduction gear angles*

necessary. Micromotor units can provide a reliable source of power in a straight low-speed handpiece. Burs can be used with an external water source, and prophy angles can be attached, as well. Some units are even combined with an ultrasonic scaler, forming a fairly complete system (Figure 9.6).

Power Scaling

Three basic types of power equipment are utilized for calculus removal: the ultrasonic, sonic, and rotary-type scalers. *Ultrasonic dental scalers,* as the name implies, operate at a frequency greater than 20 kHz. Most operate in a range of 25 kHz to 45 kHz. These scalers are popular in veterinary dentistry and are available in three types: magnetostrictive (25 kHz to 30 kHz, figure-eight tip action), piezoelectric (45 kHz, linear tip action), and ferromagnetostrictive (42 kHz, circular tip action). In general, the tips should be used parallel to the tooth and not at a right angle, to maximize the tip action and minimize tooth damage. The circular motion and high frequency decrease the working time and potential damage. Because these tips vibrate at such high frequencies, they also can generate significant heat and are cooled by a steady stream of water. Even with the water cooling, the stack-type (magnetostrictive) tips can create enough heat to result in thermal damage to the pulp if left in contact with a tooth surface for too long, in addition to potential damage from the ultrasonic frequency. Newer, thinner tips for ultrasonic scalers are available that can be used subgingivally for calculus removal below the gumline, some of which can deliver water and antimicrobial solutions directly down the tip.

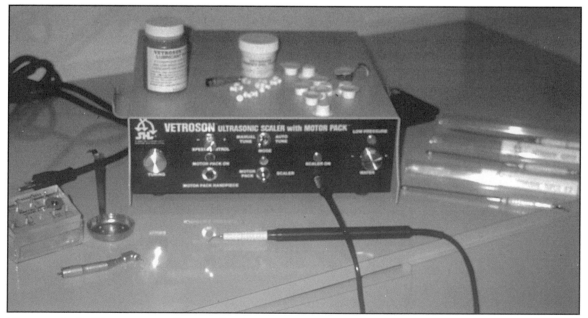

Figure 9.6 *Vetroson scaler and micromotor pack combination (Summit Hill, Navesink, NJ)*

Sonic scalers operate below 20 kHz. These are usually air driven and also irrigated with water at the tip, but because sonic scalers do not generate as much heat as ultrasonic scalers, the water is primarily used for flushing debris away for better visualization of the working area. Sonic scalers work best with adequate air pressure (30 to 40 psi at the working end). Rotary scaling is another effective way to remove calculus. A high-speed handpiece with a special six-sided *rotary bur* is used to chip away the calculus. This type of scaling; however, is very technique sensitive and could potentially damage the tooth surface if done improperly. The many forms of power scaling are quick and effective methods for calculus removal and have become popular in veterinary dentistry, given the large amounts of calculus often encountered. Yet as effective as the instruments are, they also have the potential to be detrimental and should be used according to manufacturers' recommendations.

To remain effective, the various pieces of equipment require regular maintenance with lubrication and cleaning. If the stacks of the magnetostrictive ultrasonic scalers start to splay or fracture, they need to be replaced. All tips should be examined regularly for water flow and stability. Piezoelectric tips can fatigue more quickly but are less expensive to replace than the magnetostrictive stack. The ferroceramic rod on the ferromagnetostrictive scaler can break easily if dropped and may need replacement. Sonic scalers need regular lubrication and maintenance because they can be expensive to replace. Rotary burs need to be replaced on a regular basis, as soon as the bur begins to get dull, and the operator must remember to use a lighter touch when switching to a new, sharp bur.

Polishing

Once clean, the teeth are polished to help smooth any irregularities in the outer surface of the enamel. The low-speed (less than 3,000 rpm) handpiece, prophy angle, and rubber cup are utilized, along with various prophy pastes, to polish the surface of the teeth. The prophy angle may have a latch-on, screw-on, or snap-on attachment for the rubber prophy cup. The cups come in a variety of sizes and shapes, but in general, a soft rubber cup is sufficient. Polishing, too, can generate heat if the spinning prophy cup is held in contact with the tooth surface for too long. Therefore, a light touch, gently splaying the edges of the cup as it moves across the surface of the tooth, will do. Another way to minimize the chance of thermal damage is to use sufficient prophy paste to allow the rubber cup to easily slide over the tooth. Various pastes are available, from coarse to medium to fine grit. Like sandpaper, the more coarse the grit is in the polish, the more enamel surface is removed and the more abrasive the polish. Fine-grit polish is preferred in most situations for polishing normal enamel because the coarser polishes can remove or abrade more surface than necessary.

Home Care

Once the teeth have been cleaned and polished, the best way to maintain oral health is with consistent home care. Soft-bristle toothbrushes and finger cot brushes are used to deliver specially formulated veterinary dentifrices and toothpastes. Antibacterial gels, rinses, and slow-release patches are also available. In many cases of periodontal disease, antibiotics are indicated to help decrease the bacterial population during the healing period, either in the form of oral medication or sustained release doxycycline in a gel placed into periodontal pockets. These media all help control the bacterial population associated with plaque. Daily brushing is recommended, which also helps to mechanically remove plaque.

ORAL SURGERY

Many of the instruments used for oral surgery are the same or similar to those used in general soft-tissue and orthopedic surgery, with the exception of those used for extraction purposes. For example, scalpel handles, blades (i.e., #10, 15, and 15c), Brown Adson forceps, periosteal elevators, and straight and curved scissors can all be helpful when performing oral surgery. Orthopedic wires, rasps, and acrylics are also utilized.

Extraction

For extraction purposes, the more commonly used instruments are dental elevators, *dental luxators,* and extraction forceps. Dental elevators are used to wedge between the tooth and alveolar bone or other tooth section to apply force to fatigue the periodontal ligament and "elevate" the tooth out of the alveolus, or bony socket. Smaller elevators fit the roots of cats' and small dogs' teeth, as well as deciduous teeth, and larger models are helpful with the bigger patients (Figure 9.7). Dental luxators are used to place between the root and bone in an attempt to cut the periodontal ligament. Once the periodontal ligament has been fatigued or cut, the tooth becomes loose and can be removed with the extraction forceps. Smaller forceps help minimize the temptation to use excessive force. In multirooted teeth, removal is facilitated by cutting or sectioning the tooth to remove each root individually. Tooth-cutting forceps should be used with great care to avoid fracturing the tooth or jaw. Using the high-speed handpiece and various burs (round #$1/2$ to 4 or cross-cut fissure #699, 700, or 701L), the operator can section the tooth from the furcation to the crown, creating individual root sections that are generally easier to remove. These burs and diamond discs also can be used with a low-speed handpiece, but care must be taken not to damage surrounding tissues or the operator, and an external source of coolant water must be applied (dripped from a syringe). Gigli wire can be placed through the furcation and used to cut the tooth, but because open furcations are not always present, this technique is not consistently applicable.

Various medicaments can also be placed into the socket or alveolus to help maintain a blood clot, fight infection, or help reform bone for support. Some examples include tetracycline powder, collagen, ADD (THM Biomedical, Duluth, MN), tricalcium phosphate (Peri-Oss,Miter, Warsaw, IN), calcium products, and

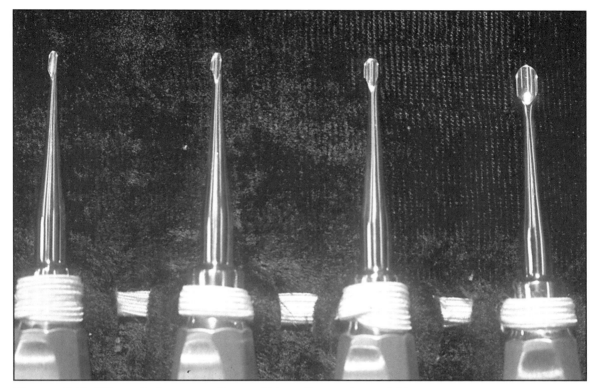

Figure 9.7 *Winged elevators (DentalAire, Santa Ana, CA)*

Consil (Nutramax, Baltimore, MD), which is a relatively new osteogenic compound. Absorbable natural or synthetic sutures can also be used to close the gingiva to help retain the medicaments and aid healing. Other oral surgeries such
as mass removals, biopsies, maxillectomies, and mandibulectomies call for more
traditional surgery packs commonly found in veterinary hospitals.

RADIOGRAPHY

The accurate diagnosis of periodontal disease, tooth structure, pathology,
and bone support is enhanced with oral radiographs. Extraoral and intraoral
radiography can provide valuable information that may otherwise go
unnoticed. Radiographic machines, films, and processing equipment are essential tools for developing and producing quality radiographs.

Extraoral Radiography

For most extraoral radiography (film outside the oral cavity), standard
X-ray machines, cassettes, and films are used to capture images such as entire
skulls, whole views of the maxilla or mandible, and temporomandibular joints.

Although certain teeth and roots can be visualized with standard machines, cassettes, and film, greater detail and isolation of individual teeth is accomplished by using intraoral film (placed inside the oral cavity).

Intraoral Radiography

Standard screens and cassettes can be placed in certain areas of the mouth, but intraoral film is much easier to place into tight areas, and it provides greater detail. Intraoral film is available in #0, 1, 2, 3, and 4 sizes, with size #0 being the smallest and size #4 the largest. Sizes #2 and 4 are the most commonly used, and they seem to be the most versatile for all situations. These are nonscreen film and therefore require more radiation for exposure, but they also provide greater detail. Standard radiographic machines can be used with the intraoral film mentioned previously, but they must be adjusted to create consistent-quality radiographs. The standard machine can be used if you can adjust the focal distance to approximately 12 inches, achieved either by lowering the tube head (the easiest method) or elevating the patient. Once the focal distance is attained, using a 100-mA setting, at 0.1 second, and with the kVp at 65 to 75, the film is placed below the structure to be radiographed and then exposed. This method will suffice but can become tedious and difficult, especially with large-breed dogs. Dental radiographic machines make this process quicker and more convenient and help reduce radiation exposure to the patient and operator. These machines are very versatile and can be maneuvered easily into proper alignment, creating more consistent results.

To develop intraoral films, standard dip tanks can be utilized following the same guidelines as if developing film from a cassette. Another way is to use rapid processing developer and fixer in small containers in the darkroom to develop the film more quickly. Various clips or hemostats are used to hold the film and dip it into the solutions, producing a radiograph usually in less than 1 minute. Operatory room or chairside developers are available to increase convenience and reduce time. These chairside developers are either automatic or consist of a box with ports to allow the operator's hands into the lightproof box and a safety shield that allows the operator to see into the box without exposing the developing film. This equipment allows the veterinary dentist to process larger quantities of film in less time and without leaving the patient's side.

RESTORATIVE DENTISTRY

Restorative, or operative, dentistry is the process of returning a tooth's structure and function. Basic materials needed for this are cavity preparation instruments, bonding agents, filling materials, prosthetic devices (such as crowns), and contouring and polishing devices. Defects in the tooth structure, whether traumatic, pathologic, or iatrogenic, ideally should be repaired to maintain the functional capacity of that tooth.

Hand Instruments

Cavity preparation can be accomplished with hand or mechanical instruments, such as burs and abrasive stones. Common burs used for cavity preparation include round, inverted cone burs and pear-shaped burs. These are used to debride cavities, smooth and contour edges or margins, and form undercuts in the cavity for better retention of fillings.

Bonding and Filling Materials

Bonding agents are cements used to enhance the seal and attachment of the filling to the dentin and enamel within the cavity. Filling materials include *amalgam,* composites, and glass ionomers. Each material has advantages and disadvantages, and each may be of more benefit in certain situations. Amalgam is considered the strongest of these. It resists wear and compression and is therefore indicated for areas known to have pressure applied, such as the occlusal surfaces of molars. Composites have the advantage of being able to be pigmented to various levels of white to match tooth shades, and for this reason, they are often chosen for defects that can be seen. Newer composites are becoming more compression resistant, increasing their popularity, and because of this, they may be used to replace amalgam. Glass ionomers do not have the compressive strength in general that composites and amalgam possess, but they have the advantage of bonding to enamel and dentin very well, creating a tighter seal within the defect. These also have the advantage of releasing fluoride over a period of time and may be beneficial for this reason. Some of the composites and glass ionomers require light activation to begin the hardening or curing process. This allows for a prolonged working time initially to adjust the filling and shape the restoration. The light activation is accomplished with a light-curing gun, which emits a high-intensity light that activates the restorative and instantly hardens it. Due to its intensity, however, this light can be damaging to the eyes of the operator or bystanders and should not be looked at directly but instead viewed through a special light-protective shield. Other products are self-curing and do not require special curing lights, but they take longer to finish.

Crowns, bridges, inlays, and onlays also fall into the category of restoratives and can all be used to restore structure and function to teeth. Crowns are available in various forms of metals or ceramics, each with advantages and disadvantages. Other equipment utilized in restorations include finishing burs, polishing disks, and stones in an assortment of sizes and shapes for contouring fillings or tooth surfaces and for finishing or smoothing areas to help retard plaque and calculus.

ENDODONTICS

Endodontic therapy requires a wide array of specialized instrumentation. In this section, the instrumentation for standard root canal therapy will be covered, as well as instrumentation and procedures for vital pulpotomy, which is within the realm of most general practice veterinarians. Root canal therapy can be broken down into three important divisions known as the "endodontic triad": preparation, sterilization, and obturation (filling). Accordingly, the instruments will be grouped into these three categories; however, some may be involved in more than one category. The vital pulpotomy procedure instrumentation was covered in more detail to give the general practitioner the basic background to perform this procedure (see chapter 5: Advanced Oral and Dental Problems—Vital Pulpotomy and Pulp Capping).

Preparation

The first step in root canal treatment is preparation. This includes opening access to the canal, removing the contents of the pulp, and cleaning and shaping the canal. Instruments used for access include the high-speed handpiece, various burs (i.e., round, pear-shaped, or inverted cone), and the root canal explorer (endodontic explorer), which is a very small-diameter metal instrument used to locate small canals. Removal of the pulp contents can be accomplished mechanically with a barbed broach, which is a notched metal shaft instrument that entangles the pulp when in the canal and is then retrieved. Some pulp removal can be done during the filing (cleaning and shaping), along with agents such as R.C.Prep (Premier Dental Co., Norristown, PA), which helps with chemical dissolution of pulp remnants. R.C.Prep is also used for its lubrication properties, allowing the files to function more efficiently. Most canal cleaning and shaping is done with files such as K-reamers, K-files, and Hedstrom files. Peeso reamers and Gates-Glidden drills are also used for this purpose but are primarily reserved for shaping the coronal one-third of the canal. The files are supplied in various widths, and the canal is filed with increasing diameters until clean, as indicated by obtaining clean white dentinal wall shavings. Other supplies helpful in these steps include: endodontic stops, endodontic organizers to organize files, an endodontic ruler to measure the depth of the canal, a bead sterilizer to sterilize files prior to use, irrigating syringe and needle, sodium hypochlorite (bleach), and sterile saline.

Sterilization

Sterilization of the canal is primarily accomplished through the actions of sodium hypochlorite (bleach) either in a nondiluted form or in a 1:1 mixture with water. This solution is used as a flush of the canal to remove debris and sterilize the canal. Care must be taken to protect the soft tissue of the oral cavity from chemical irritation and to avoid the use of sodium hypochlorite in teeth with open apexes.

Obturation (Filling)

Obturation of the canal involves lining the canal with an endodontic cement, completing the fill with a form of gutta percha, and restoring the endodontic access. Zinc oxide powder and liquid eugenol (sealer cement) is mixed on a glass slab with a spatula, then placed in the canal either with a file or with a specialized instrument called a lentulo filler. Other brand-name endodontic cements include AH-26 (Harry J. Bosworth Co., Skokie, IL) and Sealapex (Kerr Manufacturing Co., Romulus, MI). Once the canal cement is placed, the gutta percha is placed to fill the majority of the canal. Gutta percha may be used in the form of small conical points, or a heated or semisoft form may be used. The access opening is then filled with a restoration. Radiographs are also a vital component of endodontics, so the materials discussed earlier in the radiography section would be required.

Vital Pulpotomy

The equipment needed for a vital pulpotomy can be obtained at little expense, and this procedure is one you should be able to provide for your patients. The vital pulpotomy is indicated for mature tooth fractures with the pulp exposed for less than 48 hours (or immature teeth of less than 18 months with exposure less than 2 weeks), and it is intended to maintain the health of the tooth. This procedure should be performed as a sterile surgery; therefore, the area should be prepped, and sterilized instruments should be used. Materials and equipment needed include a means to remove the inflamed pulp, calcium hydroxide powder and paste, and restorative materials (see chapter 5: Advanced Oral and Dental Problems—Vital Pulpotomy and Pulp Capping).

References and Recommended

Numerous texts, both veterinary and dental, are available to supplement your knowledge of the more general subjects, such as anesthesia, surgery, and equipment. In addition, there are a number of excellent veterinary dental texts that cover all aspects of dentistry in much greater detail. A selected list of materials follows.

Crossley, C.A., and S. Penman, eds. 1995. *Manual of Small Animal Dentistry,* 2nd ed. Gloucestershire, United Kingdom: British Small Animal Veterinary Association. (Available through Iowa State University Press, 2121 S. State Ave., Ames, IA 50014-8300.)

Harvey, C.E., guest ed. 1992. Feline Dentistry. *Vet. Clinics of N. America* 22 (6).

Harvey, C.E., and P.P. Emily. 1993. *Small Animal Dentistry.* St. Louis: Mosby.

Holmstrom, S.E., guest ed. 1998. Canine Dentistry. *Vet. Clinics of N. America* 28 (5).

Holmstrom, S.E., P. Frost, and E.E. Eisner. 1998. *Veterinary Dental Techniques,* 2nd ed. Philadelphia: W.B. Saunders.

Journal of Veterinary Dentistry. American Veterinary Dental Society (1-800-322-AVDS).

Mulligan, T.W., M.S. Aller, and C.A. Williams. 1998. *Atlas of Canine and Feline Dental Radiography.* Trenton, NJ: Veterinary Learning Systems.

Wiggs, R.B., and H.B. Lobprise. 1997. Veterinary Dentistry: Principles and *Practice. Philadelphia: Lippincott-Raven.*

Glossary

— A —

Abrasion Mechanical wearing away of teeth by abnormal stresses from externally applied forces or objects. Abrasion can result from tooth-brushing habits or other abnormal stresses on the teeth.

Acanthomatous epulis A benign but locally aggressive epulis that can even infiltrate into bone. Also known as *acanthomatous ameloblast, adamantinoma,* or *basal cell carcinoma.*

Acrylic Plastics—basically methyl methacrylate mixed from a powder (polymer) and liquid (monomer)—that were once used extensively as restoratives.

Alignment Arrangement of teeth in a row.

Alveolar bone Bone that forms the sockets for the teeth.

Alveolar crest Highest part of the alveolar bone closest to the cervical line of the tooth.

Alveolar juga Bulges on the facial surface of the alveolar bone that outline the position of the roots.

Alveolar ridge The bony ridge formed by the alveolar process of the mandible and maxilla. May reduce in size when teeth are lost and functional demand for support is reduced.

Alveolar socket The cavity in the alveolar process in which the tooth root is held in place by the periodontal ligament.

Alveolus Cavity, or socket, in the alveolar process in which the root of the tooth is held.

Amalgam An alloy or combination of finely powdered metals that are mixed, or triturated, with mercury to "wet" the particles and form a condensable mass.

Ameloblast Enamel-forming cell that arises from oral ectoderm.

177

Ameloblastoma The most common tumor of the dental laminar epithelium. Slow-growing but often shows a multiple-cystic structure and can extend into bone.

Anachoresis Exposure to bacteria through a hematogenous route.

Anchorage Site of delivery from which force is exerted.

Anisognathous Unequal jaws, in which the mandibular molar occlusal zone is narrower than the maxillary counterpart; as seen in the feline, canine, bovine, equine, etc.

Ankylosis Fusion of the cementum of a tooth with alveolar bone.

Anodontia Condition in which most or all the teeth are congenitally absent.

Anterior Situated in front of; a term commonly used in reference to the incisor and canine teeth or the area toward the front of the mouth.

Anterior crossbites Classically thought of as a subclassification of Class I malocclusions but actually can be seen in Classes I, II, III, or IV. It is a condition in which cusps of one or more anterior teeth (incisors and cuspids) exceed the normal cusp relationship of the teeth in the opposing arch, labially or lingually.

Apex The terminal end or tip of a root.

Apexification The physiologic process of the apex being closed with a hard-tissue closure by action of cementoblasts and odontoblasts.

Apexogenesis Continued maturation and closure of an immature root.

Apical A direction toward the root tip or away from the incisal or occlusal surfaces.

Apical delta Multiple openings through which vessels, nerves, or other structures pass into the tooth at the apex.

Apically repositioned flap Gingival flap attached in a position more apical than its original site, often to reduce pocket depth.

Aradicular hypsodont (Subdivision of hypsodont–long-rooted.) Dentition without true roots, sometimes called open-rooted, that produces additional crown throughout life. As teeth are worn down, new crown emerges from the continually growing teeth, as seen in lagomorphs and in the incisors of rodents.

Arch See *Dental arch.*

Atraumatic malocclusion Results from genetic malpositioning of teeth or dietary causes of insufficient attrition.

Attached gingiva Tightly adherent gingiva that extends from free gingiva to alveolar mucosa.

Attrition Process of normal wear on the crown, usually caused by mastication or chewing, can be excessive.

Avulsion Tearing away of a part, such as a tooth.

— B —

Base narrow Condition in which one or both of the mandibular canines are tipped too far lingually, or toward the tongue, resulting in the cusp tip(s) making contact with the palate.

Bird tongue See *Microglossia.*

Bisecting angle technique Technique of taking radiographs to minimize linear distortion by aiming the beam perpendicularly to the line that bisects the angle formed by the long axis of the tooth and the film.

Body of the mandible Horizontal portion of the mandible, excluding the alveolar process.

Brachycephalics Individuals with short, broad facial profiles, such as boxers and bulldogs.

Brachyodont Animals whose teeth have a shorter crown-to-root ratio. Examples include primates, dogs, cats, and carnivores in general.

Buccal Pertaining to the cheek; toward the cheek or next to the cheek. Also called *facial.*

— C —

Cage-biter's syndrome Any condition that initially results in excessive attritional wear of the distal surface of a tooth.

Calcification Process by which organic tissue becomes hardened by a deposit of calcium salts within its substance. The term, in a literal sense, connotes the deposition of any mineral salts that contribute to the hardening and maturation of tissue.

Calculus Mineralized dental plaque that adheres to tooth surfaces and prosthetic dental materials.

Canal Long, tubular opening through a bone or tooth root.

Canine See *Cuspid*.

Caries Condition of decay, usually applied to teeth. *Carious* or *caries* refers to the classical black cavity with a more rapid demineralization of the dentin.

Carnassial teeth The largest shearing teeth in the upper and lower jaws (upper fourth premolar and lower first molar in the dog and cat).

Caudal infraorbital block Intraoral regional anesthetic nerve block made by injecting the infraorbital nerve at the caudal aspect of the infraorbital canal.

Cavity preparation A surgical operation that removes the caries and excises hard tissue in order to shape the tooth to receive and retain the restoration.

Cement Used to apply orthodontic brackets, appliances, crowns, or other prosthodontic devices.

Cementoblasts Cells that form cementum.

Cementoenamel junction (CEJ) Junction of enamel of the crown and cementum of the root. Also known as *cervical line*.

Cementum Layer of bonelike tissue covering the root of the tooth.

Cervical (neck, cervix) That portion of a tooth at the junction of the anatomical crown and anatomical root.

Cervical line A line formed by the junction of enamel and cementum of a tooth. Also known as *cementoenamel junction*.

Chairside developer A lightproof box with a light-selective, see-through cover in which to develop films in the operatory.

Cheeks The lateral boundary of the oral cavity.

Cheilitis Inflammation of the lips.

Cheiloschisis See *Cleft lip*.

Chlorhexidine digluconate Solution used in the treatment of periodontal disease that inhibits the development of plaque, calculus, and the onset of gingivitis in humans.

Chronic or active periodontal abscess Acute exacerbation of a chronic lesion.

Chronic Ulcerative Paradental Stomatitis (CUPS) A marked ulceration of the buccal or lingual mucosa that contact a tooth or calculus surface. Sometimes called a *kissing lesion*.

Circumferential wiring Placing wire(s) around the bone (mandible) to assist in reduction.

Cleft lip Defect or gap in the upper lip that occurs during fetal development.

Cleft palate Lack of joining together of the hard or soft palate.

Closed apex Natural constrictive closing of the tooth apex.

Closed curettage Periodontal therapy and root planing of a periodontal pocket shallow enough to reach the apical extent with hand instruments.

Commissure The junction of the upper and lower lip at the angle of the mouth.

Commisuroplasty Surgery to recontour the commissure, either to close the angle of the mouth further rostrally or to open it further.

Condyloid process Portion of the vertical ramus of the mandible that is part of the temporomandibular joint.

Coronal Toward the crown

Coronoid process Bony projection at upper anterior portion of the vertical ramus; attachment location for the temporal muscle.

Cranial infraorbital block Intraoral regional anesthetic nerve block made by injecting at the rostral end of the infraorbital canal to provide analgesia to the incisors, canines, and first two premolars.

Craniomandibular osteopathy (CMO) Enlargement of the horizontal ramus, often caudal, caused by periosteal proliferation (seen in the terrier breeds, e.g., the West Highland white terrier).

Crown That portion of a tooth, covered with enamel, that is normally visible in the oral cavity.

Crown A restorative that covers part or all of the clinical crown.

CUPS See *Chronic Ulcerative Paradental Stomatitis.*

Curette Instrument of choice for removing light subgingival calculus, root planing, and gingival and subgingival curettage.

Cusp A pronounced elevation on the occlusal surface of a tooth terminating in a conical, rounded, or flat surface.

Cuspid One of four pointed teeth, situated one on each side of each jaw, immediately distal to the corner or lateral incisors. Also known as a *canine tooth* or *fang tooth.*

— D —

Deciduous tooth A tooth that will be shed; the first dentition. Also known as a *milk tooth, primary tooth,* or *baby tooth.*

Dens-in-dente (dens invaginatus) "Tooth within a tooth," formed when the top of the tooth bud folds into itself, producing additional layers of enamel, cementum, dentin, or pulp tissue inside the tooth as it develops.

Dental arch All teeth forming an arch in either the maxilla or mandible.

Dental luxator Instrument with a wider, more delicate blade than an elevator. It is used in the periodontal space to sever the periodontal ligament attachment.

Dentigerous cyst Cystic structure arising from all or a remnant of the developing dental follicle at the neck of the tooth.

Dentin Hard, calcified tissue forming the inside body and bulk of a tooth, covered by cementum and enamel and surrounding the pulp tissue.

Dentinal bonding agents Agents that provide nearly as much bonding capacity as provided by acid-etching enamel.

Dentinal tubule Space or tube in the dentin occupied by the odontoblastic process.

Dentinoenamel junction Location within the crown of the tooth where dentin joins enamel.

Dentition General character and arrangement of the teeth, taken as a whole, as in the terms *carnivorous, herbivorous,* and *omnivorous dentition.* Primary dentition refers to deciduous teeth, secondary dentition refers to permanent teeth, and mixed dentition refers to a combination of permanent and deciduous teeth in the same dentition.

Developmental grooves Fine, depressed lines in the enamel of a tooth that mark the union of two lobes of the crown.

Diastema Any spacing between adjacent teeth in the same arch.

Dilaceration Crown or rooted structure that is bent or crooked, stemming from developmental causes.

Dimple Embossed concavity on the back side of the radiographic film, used for orientation during exposure and after development.

Distal Farthest away from the median line of the face.

— E —

Enamel Hard, calcified tissue that covers the dentin of the crown portion of a tooth.

Enamel hypocalcification A condition of poorly mineralized tooth enamel that may be soft and white to yellow to brown in color, usually because of arrested development. See *Hypocalcification*.

Envelope flap Raising of the gingiva from an underlying lesion by using a periosteal elevator at a horizontal releasing incision for exposure.

Eosinophilic granuloma complex In cats, a group of similar lesions, often with an eosinophilic component, with possible immune ramifications and some oral lesions (different types include indolent or rodent ulcers, collagenolytic granulomas, and eosinophilic plaques).

Epithelial attachment The substance produced by the reduced enamel epithelium that helps secure the attachment epithelium at the base of the gingival sulcus to the tooth.

Epulis The most common form of benign growth arising from the periodontal ligament. Three common forms found in the dog and cat are fibromatous, ossifying, or acanthomatous.

Erosion External loss of tooth hard tissue due to a chemical process without active bacterial involvement.

Eruption Movement of the tooth as it emerges through surrounding tissue so that the clinical crown gradually appears longer.

Exfoliation Shedding or loss of a primary tooth.

External resorption Loss of the outer substance of the roots, sometimes caused by traumatic forces.

Extract To pull out or remove.

Extrusion Movement of the tooth farther out of the alveolus, typically in the same direction as in normal eruption.

— F —

Facial Term used to designate the outer surfaces of the teeth collectively (buccal or labial).

Fauces Space between the left and right palatine tonsils.

Favorable fracture Mandibular fracture in a caudodorsal direction, allowing muscular forces to compress segments together.

Fibromatous epulis A fibrous form of epulis, which can be single or multiple, pedunculated or sessile.

Fibrosarcoma The third most common tumor in the dog. It is locally invasive and has a high recurrence rate but metastasizes late.

Free gingiva (free gingival margin) Gingiva that forms the gingival sulcus (marginal gingiva).

Frenulum Fold of alveolar mucosa forming a noticeable ridge of attachment between the lips and gums.

Fulcrum Center of rotation of the tooth; usually occurs approximately at the junction of the middle and apical thirds of the root.

Fully rectified current Electric current used in electrosurgery that provides easy cutting of most oral soft tissue, providing a good degree of hemostasis.

Furcation The point at which roots diverge.

Fusion tooth The result of two separate tooth buds joined at the crown by enamel and possibly dentin.

— G —

Gingiva Part of the gum tissue that immediately surrounds the teeth and alveolar bone.

Gingival hyperplasia Proliferation of the attached gingiva.

Gingival margin The crest of gingiva around the tooth.

Gingival sulcus (crevice) Subgingival space that, under normal conditions, lies between the gingival crest and the epithelial attachment.

Gingivectomy Excision of excessive gingival tissues to create a new gingival margin.

Gingivitis Inflammation involving the gingival tissues only.

Glass ionomers Compounds that chemically bind to enamel and dentin by ions forming salts that bond to the calcium in the tooth, even if slight moisture is present.

Gum-chewer's syndrome Self-trauma to the buccal mucosa and tongue caused by chewing on the tissues.

— H —

Hard palate Bony vault of the oral cavity proper covered with soft tissue.

Hemisection A tooth being cut in half, generally through the furcational area.

Heterodont Animal with more than one type (shape, size) of tooth represented in the dentition, such as incisors, cuspids, premolars, and molars. The domestic dog and cat have heterodont dentition.

High-speed handpieces Dental handpieces that provide great speed of operation but less tactile sense than low-speed handpieces. High-speed handpieces can be used for efficient removal of enamel and dentinal, bone, and other hard tissues.

Homodont Animal whose teeth are all of the same general shape or type, although tooth size may vary. Examples include fish, reptiles, and sharks.

Horizontal ramus A structure composed of the body and symphyseal area of the mandible.

— I —

Impacted Teeth not completely erupted that are fully or partially covered by bone or soft tissue.

Incisal Coronal portion or direction in incisors.

Incisive bone Rostral-most area of the upper jaw; formerly named the premaxilla. This structure accommodates the maxillary incisors and is formed solely by the medial nasal process. Also known as the *primary palate*.

Incisive foramen Foramen at the midline of the anterior palate region.

Incisive papilla Small, rounded, oblong mound of tissue directly behind or lingual to the maxillary central incisors and lying over the incisive foramen.

Incisors Central rostral teeth in either arch that are essential for cutting.

Incline plane Orthodontic appliance designed to make contact with the cusps or incisal edges of the teeth of the opposing occlusion to stimulate tooth movement directed by the incline.

Infrabony pocket Periodontal pocket whose base is apical to the alveolar crest. Also known as *intrabony pocket*.

Interarcade wiring Various mean of securing the maxilla and mandible together with wires and other implements to restrict oral movements.

Interceptive orthodontics Generally considered to be the extraction or recontouring (crown reduction) of primary or permanent teeth that are contributing to alignment problems of the permanent dentition.

Interproximal space Space between adjoining teeth.

Irreversible pulpitis Inflammation of the pulp that cannot be resolved, leading to the death of the vital pulp.

Isognathous Equal jaws, in which the premolars and molars of the opposing jaws are aligned with the occlusal surfaces facing each other and forming an occlusal plane.

— J, K, L —

Junctional epithelium Epithelium that acts to hold the mucosa in the base of the gingiva sulcus to the tooth.

Kissing lesion See *Chronic Ulcerative Paradental Stomatitis*.

Labial Next to or toward the lips.

Lamina dura Radiographic term denoting cribriform plate and bundle bone and the dense alveolar bone surrounding a root.

Lance tooth Significant mesiorostroversion of a maxillary canine.

Level bite The bite that occurs when the incisor teeth meet edge on edge or the premolars or molars occlude cusp to cusp.

Line angle Angle formed by two walls or surfaces, i.e., mesial and lingual. The junction is called the *mesiolingual line angle.*

Lingual Next to or toward the tongue.

Localized osteitis A complication caused by a combination of traumatic procedure, infection, and decreased vascular supply. It is commonly known as a *dry socket.*

Low-speed handpieces Dental handpieces with a lower speed but a highly tactile sense. These handpieces are useful for finishing, polishing, certain pin placements, and laboratory procedures.

Luxation Partial or complete dislocation from a joint, such as with the TMJ or a tooth.

— M —

Malocclusion Abnormal occlusion of the teeth.

Mandibular alveolar block Intraoral regional anesthetic nerve block made by injecting at the lingual mandible near the base of the coronoid process.

Mandibular foramen Opening on the medial surface of the ramus of the mandible for the entrance of nerves and blood vessels to the lower teeth.

Mandibular symphysis The point at which the mandibular processes merge, forming the mandible.

Mental foramen Foramen on the lateral side of the mandible, below the premolars.

Mental regional block Intraoral regional anesthetic nerve block placed at the largest mental foramen ventral to the mesial root of the second premolar. It provides analgesia to the incisors, canines, and first two premolars.

Mesial Toward or situated in the middle, for example, toward the midline of the dental arch.

Microglossia (bird tongue) A small tongue.

Mixed dentition State of having primary and permanent teeth in the dental arches at the same time.

Molars Teeth with occlusal surface that can be used to grind food or break it down into smaller pieces.

Mucogingival junction Point at which the alveolar mucosa becomes attached gingiva. Also known as *mucogingival line* or *margin*.

— N, O —

Neck Where the crown and root meet. Also known as *cervix* or *cementoenamel line*.

Occluding Contacting opposing teeth.

Occlusal Articulating or biting surface; the coronal surface of some premolars and molars.

Occlusion Relationship of the mandibular and maxillary teeth when closed or during excursive movements of the mandible; when the teeth of the mandibular arch come into contact with the teeth of the maxillary arch in any functional relationship.

Odontoblast Dentin-forming cell that originates from the dental papilla.

Odontoma A mixed odontogenic tissue tumor containing both epithelial and mesenchymal cells; either compound (disorganized mass) or complex (with denticles).

Oligodontia See *Partial anodontia.*

Open bites When a part or all of the teeth are prevented from closing to normal occlusal contact.

Open curettage Therapy and root planing of an area that has been exposed by a flap for additional visualization.

Operculum Persistence of a thick, fibrous gingiva over a partially or even fully erupted tooth.

Oral mucosa The stratified squamous epithelium that runs from the margins of the lips to the area of the tonsils and lines the oral cavity. Also known as *oral mucous membrane.*

Orthodontics That area of dentistry concerned with the supervision and guidance of the growing dentition and correction of the mature dentofacial structures. It is used to treat conditions that require movement of teeth, to correct improper relationships of the jaws and teeth, and to remedy malformations of related structures.

Osseoconductive A product that aids in the regeneration of new bone in an osseous site (as do almost all the GTR products).

Osseous wiring Placing wire(s) in direct contact with bone to provide reduction and support to segments of a bony fracture.

— P —

Palatal Pertaining to the palate, or roof of the mouth.

Palatal surface The lingual (medial) surface of maxillary teeth.

Palate The roof of the mouth.

Parallel technique Method of taking radiographs that gives the most accurate representation of proper tooth dimensions by keeping the film and the object as parallel as possible.

Partial anodontia Condition in which some, but not all, of the teeth are missing.

Pedicle flap See *Sliding flap.*

Pellicle A thin film of salivary proteins found on teeth.

Periapical Around the tip of a tooth root.

Periapical abscess Active infection around the root tip or apex, with suppuration.

Periodontal Surrounding a tooth.

Periodontal disease The inflammation of the gingiva or periodontium, their active recessive alteration, or their alteration state with or without disease.

Periodontal membrane or ligament Collagen fibers attached to the teeth roots and alveolar bone, serving to attach the tooth to the bone.

Periodontal probes Flat- or round-tipped instruments that have various lengths, in millimeters, marked on them.

Periodontitis An active disease state of the periodontium.

Periodontium Supporting tissues surrounding the teeth.

Periosteum Fibrous and cellular layer that covers bones and contains cells that become osteoblasts.

Permanent teeth The final or lasting set of teeth, which are typically very durable and lasting (the opposite of deciduous teeth). Also known as *dentes permanetes.*

Persistent deciduous teeth See *Retained deciduous teeth.*

Plaque Collection of bacteria, salivary glycoproteins, and extracellular polysaccharides that adhere to the tooth surface.

Polishing The process of smoothing scaling defects in the enamel or cementum by using a pumice rubbed against the tooth.

Posterior crossbite Condition in which the cusps of a posterior tooth (premolar, molar) in one arch exceed the normal cusp relation of those in the opposing arch, buccally or lingually.

Premaxilla Bony area of the upper jaw that includes the alveolar ridge for the incisors and the area immediately behind it, in primates.

Premolars Teeth designed to help hold and carry, like cuspids, and break food down into smaller pieces, like molars. Also known as *bicuspids.*

Primary cleft Cleft of the primary palate, at the junction between the incisive bone and maxilla.

Primary dentition First set of teeth. Also known as *baby teeth, milk teeth,* or *deciduous teeth.*

Primary palate Early-developing part of the hard palate that comes from the medial nasal process and forms a v-shaped wedge of tissue that runs from the incisive foramen forward and laterally between the lateral incisors and canines of the maxilla.

Proximal Nearest, next, or immediately adjacent to; distal or mesial.

Pseudopockets "False" gingival pockets. Increased gingival height due to hyperplasia results in deeper "pocket" readings but without attachment loss.

Pulpal exposure The unnatural opening of the pulpal chamber by a pathological or a mechanical means.

Pulpal horns The extension of the area of the pulpal chamber in the coronal section of the tooth that contains the fibers of the dental pulp.

Pulpal necrosis Partial or total pulpal death.

Pulp canal Canal in the root of a tooth that leads from the apex to the pulp chamber. Under normal conditions, it contains dental pulp tissue.

Pulp cap A treatment applied to the pulp to stimulate the formation of reparative dentin.

Pulp cavity Entire cavity within the tooth, including the root canal, pulp chamber, and horns.

Pulp chamber Cavity or chamber in the center of the crown of a tooth that normally contains the major portion of the dental pulp. The pulp canals lead into the pulp chambers.

Pulp, dental Highly vascular and innervated connective tissue contained within the pulp cavity of the tooth. The dental pulp is composed of arteries, veins, nerves, connective tissues and cells, lymph tissue, and odontoblasts.

Pulpectomy The extirpation of the entire pulp.

Pulpitis Inflammation of the pulp. The condition can be reversible or irreversible.

Pulpotomy The surgical removal of a portion of the pulp in a vital tooth.

— R —

Ranula Salivary retention cyst (sialocele) located under the tongue caused by blockage of the sublingual duct or gland.

Recession Migration of the gingival crest in an apical direction, away from the crown of the tooth.

Releasing flaps Gingival flaps raised to allow additional tooth root exposure for therapy.

Reparative dentin Localized formation of dentin in response to local trauma, such as occlusal trauma or caries; dentin that forms at the tubule access once a dead tract is formed; dentin formed by differentiated mesenchymal cells that migrate from the cell-rich zone. Also known as *tertiary dentin.*

Repositioned flap Gingival flap that is sutured to a level that is different from its original position.

Resorption Physiological removal of tissues or body products, as of the roots of deciduous teeth, or of some alveolar process after the loss of the permanent teeth.

Retained deciduous teeth Deciduous teeth that have not exfoliated once their permanent counterparts have begun to erupt.

Reversible pulpitis Inflammation of the pulp that can be resolved, returning the pulp to a healthy state.

Rodent ulcer Ulcerated thickening of the upper lip at midline; a type of eosinophilic granuloma in cats. Also known as *indolent* ("not painful") *ulcer.*

Root That portion of a tooth normally embedded in the alveolar process and covered with cementum.

Root canal See *Pulp canal.*

Root exposure Uncovering or exposure of the root surfaces caused by periodontal tissue loss.

Root planing Process of smoothing the cementum of the root of a tooth.

Root resection The cutting off of a root but not its associated portion of crown.

Rotary bur Six-sided, noncutting, soft-steel bur that utilizes the high-speed handpiece on an air-driven unit and reaches a frequency of about 30 kHz.

Rubber jaw Soft, flexible jaw structure caused by depletion or loss of calcium.

Rugae Small ridges of tissue extending laterally across the anterior of the hard palate.

— S —

Salivary glands Glandular system secreting saliva, a serous and mucous fluid that assists in the lubrication and digestion of food.

Scissor bite The normal relationship of the maxillary incisors overlapping the mandibular incisors whose incisal edges rest on or near the cingulum on the lingual surfaces on the maxillary incisors.

Secondary cleft Palatal cleft of the secondary palate, i.e., on the midline.

Sharpey's fibers Part of the periodontal ligament, embedded in cementum or alveolar bone.

Shed Term used for the exfoliation of deciduous teeth.

Sialocele Retention cyst of salivary fluids.

Sliding (pedicle) flap Flap or graft of attached gingiva harvested from a site adjacent to a defect and rotated on its base once incised to cover the defect.

Soft palate The unsupported soft tissue that extends back from the hard palate, free of the support of the palatine bone.

Sonic (subsonic) scalers Scalers that operate by compressed gas or air pressure, creating an oval-elliptical tip oscillation generally at less than 20 kHz.

Stomatitis Inflammation of the soft tissues of the oral cavity or mouth.

Straight handpiece Handpiece used in standard dental procedures that usually generates 6,000 rpm.

Strategic teeth Teeth that may be important to the animal's well-being, usually the cuspids and the carnassials.

Subgingival calculus scaling Removal of subgingival deposits of calculus.

Subgingival curettage Removal of diseased soft tissue within a periodontal pocket.

Subgingival debridement Moderate scaling or gentle root planing and soft-tissue debridement of subgingival areas.

Subluxation Incomplete dislocation of a joint, such as the TMJ, or of a tooth.

Submerged teeth Teeth covered by bone.

Sulcus See *Gingival sulcus.*

Supernumerary teeth Those teeth beyond the normal complement; extra teeth.

Suprabony pocket Periodontal pocket with its base, or bottom, coronal to the alveolar crestal bone.

— T —

Temporomandibular joint (TMJ) The joint made of the condylar process of the vertical ramus of the mandible and the mandibular fossa of the temporal bone of the skull.

Tight lip Condition in which the lower lip has a deficient vestibule, causing the lip to ride over the mandibular incisors and even canines. It is most commonly seen in the Chinese shar pei.

Tooth eruption The emergence and movement of the crown of the tooth into the oral cavity.

Tooth resection The cutting off of a portion of the crown, with or without its associated root structure.

Transillumination Assessment of the reflectivity of the internal tooth structure to evaluate vitality of the pulp by placing a light behind a tooth and viewing it.

Transosseous wiring Placing wire(s) across a fracture line incorporating the segments for stabilization.

— U Through Z —

Ultrasonic dental scalers Dental scaling instruments functioning at greater than 20 kHz. These instruments work by two basic principles, mechanical kick and cavitation. Mechanical kick is the actual effect of the metal tip contacting the calculus, while the water spray hitting the vibrating tip is energized to cavitate or clean the tooth surface.

Underbite A term loosely applied to certain divisions of Class I and III malocclusions but most typically applied to Class III malocclusions.

Unfavorable fracture Mandibular fracture running caudoventrally, with muscular forces able to distract the segments.

Varnish Protective material that keeps chemical irritants from the pulp, as well as providing marginal seals to reduce microleakage.

Vertical releasing incisions Incisions made at the mesial and distal aspects of the horizontal releasing incision for a full releasing flap.

Vestibule Space between the lips or cheeks and the teeth.

Wry mouth Condition in which one of the four jaw quadrants is grossly out of proportion to the other three, causing a facial deviation from the midline.

Zinc ascorbate Solutions that have been shown to support collagen synthesis and generally reduce bad breath for a short period.

Zygomatic arch Arch of bone on the side of the face or skull formed by the zygomatic bone and temporal bone.

Periodontitis, 40, 191; early, 43;
    juvenile, 45, 137; refractory, 45;
    severe, 44-45
Periodontium, 9-10, 41, 191
Periosteal elevator, 85, 161, 168
Periosteal flap: elevation of, 91 (fig.);
    placement of, 91 (fig.);
    suturing, 92 (fig.)
Periosteum, 75, 191
Persistent deciduous teeth. *See*
    Retained deciduous teeth
Pharyngitis, 12, 70 (photo)
Planing: closed-root, 52, 53 (photo);
    flap, 55 (photo); open-root, 55
    (photo); root, 43, 49, 52, 193
Plaque, 12, 191; intolerance, 45, 140;
    removing, 43, 162-63, 168
Plate stabilization, 128 (photo)
Pockets: infrabony, 40, 44, 52, 56,
    187; palatal, 58 (photo);
    periodontal, 137, 139; therapy,
    44; up to 5 mm, 52-54; up to 9
    mm, 54-57
Polishing, 49, 167, 191; improper, 51
Posterior crossbite, 99, 104, 105
    (photo), 191
Posterior teeth, 158; in
    rodents/lagomorphs, extracting,
    160
Power instruments, 164, 166-67; for
    calculus removal, 162, 166
Preanesthetic workups, 49
Premaxilla, 191
Premolars, 2, 191; pinking-shear
    configuration for, 9; unerupted/
    embedded, 26 (photo)
Primary cleft, 34 (photo), 191
Primary dentition, 191
Prophy angles, 94, 164 (photo), 165
    (photo), 166
Prophylaxis, 42, 47, 49-52, 61;
    instruments for, 162; routine,
    48
Prophy paste, 51, 167
Prosthodontics, 113

Proximal, 192
Pseudopockets, 29, 192
Pulp, 192; anatomy, 6-7; endontically
    compromised, 95; nonvital, 94,
    95, 97; removal of, 97;
    vessels/nerves, 7
Pulpal exposure, 143, 192
Pulpal horns, 7, 192
Pulpal necrosis, 192
Pulp canal, 192; exposure of, 93-94
Pulp capping, 95, 96, 105, 192
Pulp cavity, 6-7, 142, 192
Pulp chamber, 7, 192
Pulpectomy, 192
Pulpitis, 12, 94-95, 192; problems
    with, 27; reversible/
    irreversible, 63 (photo), 120,
    187, 193; treatment options for,
    95
Pulpotomy, 192; vital, 95, 96, 96 (fig.),
    101, 173

Rabbits, dental formula of, 151
Radiographs, 19, 22, 74, 75, 96, 113,
    146, 151, 170; detail on, 15;
    emergency, 116; endodontics
    and, 173; extraoral, 14;
    intraoral, 15-16, 75, 141, 152,
    161, 161 (photo), 170;
    postoperative, 24, 82
Radiography, 14-17, 19, 21-24, 49, 52,
    131; external, 169-70;
    materials/equipment for, 161,
    169-70; technique for, 16-17
Ranula, 34-35, 193; sublingual, 35
    (photo)
Rasps, 159 (photo), 168
Rats, dental formula of, 150-51
R.C. Prep, 172
Reamers: K-, 172; Peeso, 172
Recession, 193
Reduction gear angles, 164, 165
    (photo)
Regenerative therapy, 49, 55-57
Reimplantation, tooth, 123

About the Authors

Heidi Bachmann Lobprise is a 1983 graduate of Texas A & M University and has been an associate at the Dallas Dental Service Animal Clinic since 1987. She completed her veterinary dental residency with Robert Wiggs in 1992 and passed the AVDC examination to become a diplomate of the American Veterinary Dental College in 1993. She is the immediate past president of the American Veterinary Dental Society and is coauthor of *Veterinary Dentistry— Principles and Practice.*

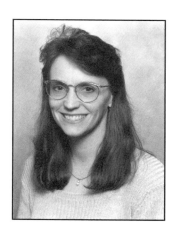

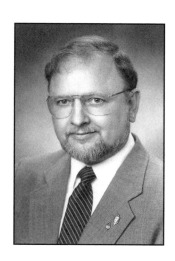

Robert B. Wiggs is a 1973 graduate of Texas A & M University College of Veterinary Medicine. He has practiced in the Dallas area since graduation and started a career-long interest in veterinary dentistry in college. He was one of the first members of the American Veterinary Dental Society and a charter Fellow of the Academy of Veterinary Dentistry; he also passed the first examination of the American Veterinary Dental College (AVDC) to become a diplomate in 1989. He is a past president of the American Veterinary Dental Society and was the key spokesperson for several years for the National Pet Dental Health Month's "Pets Need Dental Care, Too" campaign. Currently president (1998 to 2000) of the American Veterinary Dental College, he has lectured extensively around the world and is the author of numerous publications and articles, including *Veterinary Dentistry—Principles and Practice.*